SONG FOR ROSALEEN

PIP DESMOND

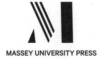

MASSEY UNIVERSITY PRESS

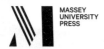

MASSEY
UNIVERSITY
PRESS

First published in 2018 by Massey University Press
Private Bag 102904, North Shore Mail Centre
Auckland 0745, New Zealand
www.masseypress.ac.nz

Text and images copyright © Pip Desmond, 2018
Cover image copyright © Shutterstock

Design by Kate Barraclough

A catalogue record for this book is available from the
National Library of New Zealand

Printed and bound in China by Everbest Ltd

ISBN: 978-0-9951001-2-1
eISBN: 978-0-9951001-3-8

For Mum

'Have you asked her if you can write about her?' said my writer friend.
  'She's dead.'
  'I know. But have you asked her?'
  'I'm scared she'll say no.'
  Before I could pluck up the courage, Mum came to me in a dream, wading out of a lake, the hem of her skirt dragging in the mud. 'You haven't forgotten about me, have you?' she said.

Do not go gentle into that good night,
Old age should burn and rave at close of day;
Rage, rage against the dying of the light.
— Dylan Thomas

CONTENTS

1. Speaking out _____ 7
2. Tamarillo chutney _____ 16
3. Babies _____ 27
4. Portfolios _____ 36
5. Wonderland _____ 45
6. Circle the wagons _____ 53
7. Different mothers _____ 64
8. Silver weddings _____ 76
9. Driving test _____ 84
10. Therapeutic fibbing _____ 92
11. Role models _____ 100
12. Wise old woman _____ 109
13. Ladylike behaviour ____ 120
14. Hair cuts _____ 133
15. Party over _____ 138
16. Boarding school blues __ 147

17. A new friend _____ 158
18. Home visit _____ 169
19. A prayer _____ 177
20. Acts of kindness _____ 184
21. Alive inside _____ 190
22. The star _____ 199
23. Hole in the hallway ____ 206
24. Toothache _____ 214
25. Alone is lonely _____ 223
26. Fortisip _____ 232
27. Going home _____ 239

Epilogue _____ 247
Bibliography _____ 252
Acknowledgements ____ 253
About the author _____ 255

CHAPTER ONE

SPEAKING OUT

'WHAT'S THE ONE thing you can't say?' asked the voice at the other end of the phone.

Without warning, a picture of my mother filled my mind. She'd been dead for six years, had vascular dementia for almost as long before that. When she started forgetting, she was in her early seventies, a widow, living alone. My four sisters, brother and I rallied round her as best we could while she fought the disease she didn't know she had. It was a sad, bewildering time that tested our certainties and bonds.

The caller was from the 2015 TEDxWellingtonWomen team. Barely back on New Zealand soil from two years overseas, I'd been invited to speak at their event and was struggling to come up with a topic. Her question cut through my confusion. The one thing I couldn't say was that I still wanted to write about my mother.

I'd been wanting to write about Mum since she died. The decision seemed simple at first. It was my story to tell; Mum wasn't around to veto or be hurt by it. But it was also my siblings' story. While some supported the idea, others had misgivings. These were around keeping our mother's memory — and memory loss — sacred and intact and private. Just like Mum herself, a backroom girl, never one for the limelight.

I mostly believed that putting our experience into words would help my family and perhaps others come to terms with the heartbreak that is dementia. But I couldn't guarantee that. Memoirs tear some families apart. I had hit an impasse: my right to speak out, others' for silence. I sensed Mum's hand beyond the grave packing me off to Timor-Leste with my husband Pat for two years. Time out to cool my heels. But now we were home and her story continued to tug at my sleeve.

Delving into my past and revealing other people's lives was not new to me. While Mum had dementia, I wrote *Trust*, a book about a group of Wellington gang women with whom I'd lived and worked in the 1970s. As I struggled with my responsibilities to them and their stories, my tutor told me, 'Write as if everyone's dead and worry about people's feelings later.' Good advice for unleashing creative flow, no use for unpicking ethics.

Ethics were my focus on the wintry May afternoon that I stood in the red TEDx circle in the Wellington City Gallery, sick with terror that my mind would go blank as it had at the dress rehearsal. The thought of my daughter Megan in the 100-strong audience steadied me. I took a deep breath and projected the phrase 'Compassionate Truth' on the big screen behind me. Historian Michael King's litmus test for biographers came close to my own, I said. Yes, we must be fearless in the pursuit of truth but we must be equally compassionate towards those whose lives we trample through in search of it.

Using my gang women experience, I talked about the power of stories to heal and connect us, but also their potential to re-traumatise even willing subjects and to expose unwitting bystanders. Back and forth I went between the merits and perils of baring our souls, searching for the alchemy between truth and compassion that would make everything all right. The best I could come up with was that comparing notes as honestly as we can encourages us to stand back and reflect on our lives — and when we reflect, we find compassion, not just for other people but for ourselves.

Finally I put up a photo of Mum two years before she died, holding her great-granddaughter Avah. Mum's head is bowed over the sleeping baby, her crooked fingers cradle Avah's perfect ones. Old life greets new. I acknowledged I wanted to write about Mum and said for now I had to sit with the *don't know*. My final words were a warning: 'Proceed with caution. Lives and relationships are at stake when we decide to tell a story, even one we regard as our own.'

AS I WALKED offstage, I felt giddy with relief that my memory hadn't let me down. But beneath this euphoria was a growing clarity. The tension between speaking out and shutting up was never going to go away. Not writing about Mum wouldn't solve the angst, just shuffle it around. Somehow the answer lay in the doing of it, fraught and messy as that might be.

I already had the scaffolding for the story: thousands of emails between me and my siblings that chronicled our care of Mum after she got dementia. During this time I'd noted down some of my key conversations with her. Even more precious, I'd captured her voice on tape reminiscing about her childhood. Letting me record her memories had taken some persuading. She was a listener not a talker; she couldn't imagine why her life would interest anyone else. But when her brother Des came to visit from Adelaide in October 2003, I'd pinned them both down.

Even then she was sceptical. 'If we get a wriggle on we can be finished by lunchtime,' she said as I arrived to the smell of fresh coffee and homemade shortbread.

'I hope not,' I said. I'd put aside the whole day for this and was in no hurry to swap the tranquillity of Mum's house for the teenage-boy hubbub of my own. I set up my tape recorder at one end of her oval dining table that seated 12 at a squash. Through the sliding doors, a medley of pot plants vied for space on a narrow deck.

Des appeared and wrapped me in an awkward hug.

'Who wants to go first?' I asked when Mum had cleared the cups.

'I go first,' she said — so unlike her.

Des tipped his head in her direction. 'Yes. Oldest.' At 73, his big sister could still pull rank.

'Rosaleen Mary Desmond.' Mum gave her married name in clipped vowels, followed by her date of birth: 'Eighteen — eleven — twenty-nine. Born in Roxburgh Cottage Hospital.' Des came four years later. They had an older half-brother, Gerard, from their father's first marriage, but he was away at boarding school and didn't figure in their young lives.

As Mum and Des relaxed, a familiar tale emerged: immigrants arriving in Aotearoa New Zealand in the 1860s and 1870s in search of gold, land and a better life. On their father's side were the Waigths of German and English descent — 'austere', Mum said; on their mother's, the outgoing Kearney clan, Irish through and through. I recognised some of the names from the family tree that Mum had embroidered as a young woman, and which still hung in her lounge.

John Harry Waigth was nearly 50 when Mum was born. Orchardist, mayor of Roxburgh (like his father and brother), a pillar of the Catholic Church, he seemed more like a kindly grandfather to his two younger children. His second wife, Mary

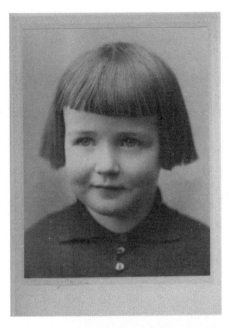

left
Mum, about
five years old.

———

below
Mum and her
brother Des,
around 1939.

———

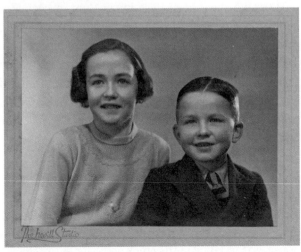

Rose, was 20 years his junior and had grown up on a sheep farm in Ranfurly.

Despite being babies of the Depression, Mum and Des had a secure and bountiful childhood in the modest brick house set in lovely grounds off the main road of the small Central Otago town. There were veges and chickens in the garden, milk delivered to metal cans at the gate, apricots and cherries from the orchard established by their grandfather. All year round the whole family slept on the open verandah, canvas blinds the only buffer against winter nights that froze sheets on the washing line and water in the pipes. 'It was a very healthy upbringing,' said Mum, who on this mild spring day in Wellington had her wood burner cranked up to sauna levels.

As the young wife of an important man, Mary Rose cooked and sewed, bottled and pickled, had a talent for flower-arranging, was on the church cleaning roster and the school committee. She didn't read much, Des said. 'She was a very proud lady, proud of her presentation. Always well dressed and her hair well done. All those Kearney girls were.'

He could have been describing Mum, except Mum usually had two books on the go, one upstairs and one for bed. I glanced across the polished table at her. In spite of her love of good food and the cream that laced her coffee, she'd become gaunt in the ten years since Dad died. But a bright lipstick offset the striped blouse buttoned to the neck to hide her wrinkles. Two gold chains hung over it, matched by discreet gold earrings. Her hair was permed, face powdered, cheeks rouged, just like every morning, visitors or not. Elegance ran in her blood, it seemed.

My fear that Des, the schoolteacher, might dominate the conversation quickly faded. Brother and sister had an easy rapport. Before my eyes, they turned back into whispering, wide-eyed children, free to play in the gum plantation behind the house, go tadpoling in the creek and bake at the swimming baths on long summer afternoons.

A cast of unconventional adults populated their lives. Foremost among these 'homegrown characters' were their mother and her sisters, Sarah and Vera. These women were not just classy dressers but forthright, spirited women, practical jokers with a strong attachment to each other.

They loved the races, Mum said. 'I can still see her' — she meant her mother — 'sitting listening to the trots over the radio, and she'd be riding.' Mum bounced up and down in her chair like a jockey, flapping her arms.

Sarah, the oldest, was partial to a port wine and brandy before lunch. To demonstrate the effect of her aunt's whisky-laced trifle on Mum's four-year-old cousin Laurette, Mum rocked back and forth before pitching headfirst into the table. I couldn't remember when I'd last seen her so animated.

I wondered if she was lonelier than she let on. After Dad's death, she'd kept going without complaint, filled her days with useful tasks, cooked nutritious meals for one and seemed to cherish her solitude. Perhaps she'd had no choice, I thought. Unlike the generations of women before and after her, Mum didn't have a safety net of sisters to fall back on. She blessed her five daughters with that gift — the complex love borne of shared genes, shared gender, shared history — but she had to walk through life alone.

Except for us, of course, her six children and 18 grandchildren. Like me, my younger sisters Rose, Ginny and Kate lived nearby. During school holidays, my older sister Liz often made the four-hour trip from Hastings with a carload of kids, while my only brother Matt yo-yoed between his work in South East Asia and family in Wellington.

But Mum needed company her own age. I was pleased that Des and his wife Chris were taking her down south to visit descendants of the relatives they'd been talking about. 'Your bloody cousins,' Des said. He was quoting his older cousin Jack, he explained at our looks of surprise: my balding, softly spoken uncle didn't usually swear.

Jack had Alzheimer's disease, Des said. 'Occasionally he and his wife went downtown to Alexandra to do some shopping, which is not very big, and when he came out, he couldn't find her or his car. Everybody was helping him to look for a yellow Holden. They eventually found her sitting in a blue Datsun.' He chuckled.

'It's not funny, Des,' Mum said quietly. 'It is when you're your age. But it's not funny at my age.'

Undeterred, Des carried on. Jack's family asked his doctor to say he wasn't fit to drive. But when Jack turned up for the medical, a locum gave him the all-clear. So his children took his car keys. The last time Des had called in, Jack thumped him on the chest and said, 'It was your bloody cousins that did it. 'Not "*my* children" but "*your* cousins",' Des said.

Everyone joined in the laughter this time, including Mum. We stopped for lunch and she produced macaroni cheese in individual ramekins out of nowhere. There was no more talk of finishing early. Once undammed, her memories flowed as deep as the Clutha River that skirted Roxburgh but was too dangerous to swim in.

When we resumed, the talk turned to boarding school, the only option for small-town Catholic kids seeking an academic and religious college education. Mum's main memories of St Dominic's College in Dunedin, 100 miles from Roxburgh, where she was one of 30 boarders, were of early homesickness, the dreadful wartime food rations, and the 'absurd' discipline of the Dominican sisters.

She pushed a faded blue magazine across the table towards me. '*The Dominican Star*, December 1947', I saw on the cover. 'You can read it later,' she said.

As the afternoon darkened, the stories began to circle back on each other. Mum was looking tired. 'I think we're all running out of puff because I feel as if Des and I are starting to get a bit boring now,' she said in her no-nonsense way. 'We probably need a port wine and brandy.'

'Will gin do?' I asked, turning off my tape recorder. I took the stopper out of the decanter on the walnut sideboard, a Roxburgh heirloom. When we all had a glass in hand, I proposed a toast to their South Island trip.

Back home I pored over Mum's school magazine, spirited away in a drawer for more than 50 years, and found her everywhere in its pages. She returned to college as a senior boarder a week late because she was 'tripping in the North Island', according to a gossipy diary entry. She took the part of Our Lady in a school play. R. Waigth topped the list of Form V 'optima students'. She won prizes for literature and history and passed an advanced senior elocution exam. Even more thrilling, she won the 'Wreath', a special prize decided by pupils. (Des later told me she won it an unprecedented two years in a row.)

But the biggest shock was finding Mum in a photo of the debating team that competed in the Bishop's Shield, a regional competition between seven Catholic colleges, boys and girls. Not only did the team win their debate but Mum was also the best speaker. I was flabbergasted. The first time I heard her make a speech was at a family birthday when she was in her seventies. While Dad was alive, she rarely ventured an opinion in public; he did the talking for both of them. I wondered when the intelligent, popular, articulate young woman in the black gym frock holding the shield had lost her voice, and whether she might be finding it again.

A week later, Mum was back from the South Island. Everything had gone well, she said. But it was good to be home.

That night, Des phoned. He came straight to the point. 'I've got bad news, Pip,' he said. 'There's something wrong with Rosaleen.'

CHAPTER TWO

———

TAMARILLO CHUTNEY

I RANG LAURETTE, Mum's favourite cousin. They'd stayed with her in Oamaru on their way south. If anything was amiss, she'd have noticed.

'We had a wonderful time,' she said. 'Sat up all night drinking gin and giggling like school girls. Just like our mothers. Dolly and Vera were as silly as chooks when they got together. They'd dress up, mix and match, giggle all the time.'

I forced myself to spell out Des's concerns: that Mum had got confused about money. That she talked over everyone when they went visiting. And she kept wandering off. She'd have ended up on the tarmac at Christchurch airport if they hadn't stopped her.

'She probably just needed a bit of space,' Laurette said. 'Three of them cooped up in that little rental car. She's got used to her own company since your father died.'

Feeling like a traitor, I blurted out Des's worst charge: that he'd found Mum's undergarments strewn along the hall after her bath. This was unthinkable. No one was more particular or private than my mother.

'Oh, she might have dropped a hanky or something.' Laurette wasn't budging. Mum was fine, just the same as ever.

I rang my sisters and gave them the all-clear. We agreed that Des had been away a long time, he didn't know Mum very well. She was in her seventies now. Older people got a bit absent-minded, especially when out of their comfort zone. Everyone knew that.

We were more worried about Mum's physical health. Her blood pressure was finally under control, but she had osteoporosis and so much joint pain that the specialist was doing tests for rheumatoid arthritis. Digging in her garden one day, she'd torn the rotator cuff of her right shoulder and was deemed too old for surgery. When she ate, she braced the injured arm against her side like a broken wing and brought her head down to meet her hand.

In spite of her ailments, Mum kept her two-storey house in Colville Street impeccable, spent hours tending her plants and pots, and cut her patch of lawn with an electric mower. She and Dad had moved into the quiet Newtown cul-de-sac in the early 1980s, ignoring their friends' tut-tutting about the suburb's unsavoury reputation — at least partly, I like to think, to be close to Pat and me and their only Wellington-based grandchildren at the time.

By then Dad had been sick for more than a decade, four of us had left home, and their sprawling, six-bedroom house in Wadestown with its steep, grassed terraces had become a burden. They looked for a long time before settling on the substantial mock-Tudor house on the other side of town, one of four being sold off the plans.

When it was built, Mum set about transforming the interior to her usual high standards. At street level, there was internal access through a double garage. The lounge had a high stud and north-facing windows that embraced the sun and a stand of native trees until developers got hold of them. 'Never let a man design a kitchen,' Mum used to say. Her own had everything within reach and was small enough to discourage people from milling about while she cooked. Downstairs were four bedrooms and a rumpus room, and upstairs a walk-in attic packed with enough stuff to set up a St Vincent de Paul shop.

It was time to downsize, we'd suggested. Find somewhere more compact, on one level, with less maintenance. It became a Sunday morning ritual. I'd line up two or three open homes and pick Mum up after she'd been to Mass. Off we'd go, poking our noses into other people's clutter, gossiping about them afterwards. We'd been doing it for months.

In a lounge in Mount Victoria that was not much wider than my outstretched arms, I waxed on about the light, the view, the polished wooden floors.

Cold in winter, Mum said. She had lots of light where she was. And where would all her furniture go?

We walked through to the kitchen. I pointed out the big pantry, she the lack of bench space. Beyond it was a tiny courtyard. Me: What a sun trap. Her: Nowhere to garden.

The real estate agent joined us. 'So what sort of place are you looking for, Mrs Desmond?'

'Ask my daughter,' Mum said. 'She's the one who wants me to move.'

ON THE WAY home we stopped at Oriental Bay for an ice cream from the dairy with 40 flavours, joining the throngs who knew better than to stay inside when the sun shone in Wellington. Spray from the fountain floated across the water. Children shrieked in the shallows and dug in the sand. Mum asked after my own kids, as she always did. I told her that Jackson, the youngest, was about to go flatting like the older two. She made approving noises about their independence — although when I left home at 19, she'd cried for a week, she told me. It wouldn't have been so bad if I'd been moving to another city or overseas like Matt and Liz. But she couldn't understand why I'd want to swap the comfort of our Wadestown home for a student dive at the bottom of the hill that she had to drive past every day to take Dad to work.

I'd already delayed my leaving for a year because of the severe epileptic seizures that blindsided my father in his mid-forties, and was desperate to flee not just the childhood cocoon but also his veiled despair and Mum's hypervigilance. I must have seemed ungrateful. She had to leave home at 13 to go to boarding school. After she married Dad, she moved even further from her mother, following him to Wellington, his home town, in the interests of his career. There'd been five houses in the capital, Colville Street the last. It was there Mum had nursed Dad and laid out his body after he died. And it was the only one she'd lived in by herself. Her whole identity was tied up in it.

'You're not really serious about shifting, are you?' I said.

Mum looked sheepish. 'I'm managing fine. And there are so many good things about where I live now.'

'I know, Mum. But that house is too big for one little old lady.'

'Seventy-something's not old,' she said. 'And I need more than a shoebox so people can come and stay.' That may have been true in the past but her standards were so high that overnight guests wore her out now. Even at the height of her hospitality, she'd been fond of saying, *Visitors are like fish: they go off in three days*. This rule never applied to her own children. All of us had decamped there between houses, countries, jobs, relationships. We brought our partners and kids, and arrived to beds smelling of fresh linen, folded towels at the ends.

When Pat and I renovated our house in the 1980s, we moved into Colville Street for three months. On weekends, Mum looked after our two pre-schoolers and sent us off with filled rolls and home baking to sustain us while we put up gib board and painted walls. It may have been the quickest way to get rid of us but it was heroic all the same. The least I could do was respect her wishes now.

'OK, no more house-hunting,' I said, as I pulled up outside her gate. 'But please don't leave it too long. Everyone agrees it's better to move before you have to.'

'Don't worry, I'll know when it's time,' she said.

I drove to the end of the street and turned around. As I passed her house, Mum waved me down. I pulled up beside her small porch adorned with hanging baskets full of petunias, busy Lizzie, black aeonium and other flowers whose names I could never remember.

She handed me two jars through the car window. 'Nearly forgot,' she said. 'It's tamarillo season. My annual batch.'

'Thanks, Mum, it's Pat's favourite.' As I drove away, I watched her through the rear vision mirror. She was still standing at the gate when I turned the corner, a hunched figure seeing me off. At home, I placed the two jars of scarlet chutney in the pantry next to the two she'd given me the week before and the two the week before that. I shut the door and tried to put them out of my mind.

MUM AND I sat in the departure lounge at Wellington airport looking at the rain beating down on the runway. Our flight to Auckland had been delayed; it was touch and go whether we'd get to her cousin's funeral on time.

'We'll still go, won't we?' Mum pleaded, like a child who fears a treat is about to be taken away. I hadn't realised how much she'd been counting on the overnight trip, a chance to see Liz who was driving up from Hawke's Bay, Laurette, and other relations; Mum usually accepted disappointment without complaint. It came as even more of a surprise that she thought the decision was in my hands.

I squeezed her thin arm. 'Yes, we'll still go,' I said.

ON A BRISK winter morning in July, Mum and I strolled along the Seatoun foreshore. She never turned down an invitation to go out, although she never initiated one either, or rang just for a chat. 'You girls are so busy,' she'd say, as if she didn't warrant taking up our time.

Our progress was slow. Mum seemed more unsteady than usual. Her legs didn't want to obey her, she said; she had to consciously lift one, then the other. I took her arm: all bone, no padding. When we came to a wooden seat, we stopped to rest and watch the waves shuffle up and down the shingly beach. Mum pointed to a path rising sharply between houses on the bush-clad hill across the road. 'Our access in Kelburn was like that,' she said. 'Boundary Road. When I went out, I had to carry you up seventy steps.' Since the day I recorded her childhood memories, she'd been bringing up the past more, as if taking the top off one memory revealed a cluster of others inside it, like Russian dolls.

The Kelburn house was their first, after Mum and Dad moved to Wellington in 1957 with four children under four: Rose only three months old. A childless friend found it for them before they arrived, Mum said. There was a housing shortage in Wellington and they were grateful. I didn't think to ask her the address but after she died, I searched the electoral roll. Sure enough, there they were: Frederick Bernard Desmond, medical practitioner; Rosaleen Mary Desmond, housewife, 19 Boundary Road.

I drove up past the university to take a look, wishing Mum was beside me. Past the Kelburn shops I turned right and parked at the bottom of a narrow, dead-end street. A concrete path disappeared into dense bush, broken by short flights of steps: I counted 50 on my way down. Eventually I came to number 19, a double-storey wooden house, grander than I'd expected, with only one visible neighbour. No one answered when I knocked. I was relieved in a way: I wasn't sure how I felt about stepping back into the past without a guide.

In Dad's version of these years, four chubby cherubs tumbled over each other from morning till night. Except that he wasn't there from morning till night: he was out in the world pursuing his twin loves of medicine and God. It was Mum who was left alone with the cherubs, two of whom didn't walk. There was no way she could have got a pushchair up that zig-zagging path and all those steps. Even if she had, it was an uphill slog to the shops and Dad took their only car to work.

Another family story — that Mum had us all in bed by 4.30 in the winter — took on a new light. It had always been cited as evidence of her efficiency. Now I wondered if it said more about her desperation. How lonely she must have been in that secluded house in a new city. Her mother, her main support, was equally bereft at the separation, Des told me. Alone in her brick house in Roxburgh, she cooked a pot of porridge and lived on nothing else for weeks.

MUM TRIPPED WHILE carrying a basket of wet clothes down a concrete step to the washing line at the back of the house, a dark corner that never saw the sun. She jarred her spine but somehow her bones survived the impact. As a precaution, her GP put her on a bone density drug called Fosamax. Mum had to take the unwieldy pill once a week, first thing in the morning, on an empty stomach. Afterwards, she wasn't allowed to lie down, eat or drink for half an hour. Every time I called in, she waved the box at me and asked me to explain the instructions again. The fall seemed to have shaken up more than her delicate frame.

If I mentioned her forgetfulness, she'd tell me everyone her age complained of the same thing. Memory like a sieve. In one ear, out the other. 'Megan's right,' she'd say, parroting my daughter: 'Grandma, you just need to concentrate.'

I offered to go with her next time she saw her GP. She seemed grateful. But when I followed her into the surgery, she glared at me and said nothing about her memory. The GP looked surprised when I brought it up. She asked Mum the prime minister's name, what city she lived in, the day of the week. Mum rattled off the answers in a reproachful voice. I felt foolish. If that was how memory problems were measured, we were clearly over-reacting.

The GP was reassuring. Pain could be very distracting, she said. The Panadeine Mum was taking after her fall contained codeine, which could affect her short-term memory. Once her physical symptoms settled down, everything else probably would too. Just to be sure, she'd refer Mum to the geriatrician at Wellington Hospital. Mum stalked out ahead of me but stayed within earshot so I couldn't whisper my concerns behind her back. We drove home in silence.

IT WAS MUM'S birthday, a year since Des's warning. Her five daughters planned a celebration for her at Rose's beach house in Waikanae, an hour away. Spending a weekend together had become a more or less annual event since Dad died. Matt was usually out of the country, leaving our female ecosystem undisturbed.

Mum phoned me around midday. She was too sick and her back was too sore to go away, she said. We couldn't abandon her.

A few quick emails, and the venue became Colville Street. We'd cheer her up with good food and wine, watch movies, make the most of the city.

After work, I let myself into Mum's house, noting she'd forgotten to lock the front door again. She was sitting in the lounge with the wood burner roaring, wheat bags draped around her neck and down her arm, Maurice Gee's *Live Bodies* spine-up on her lap. Around her were the tasteful props of a lifetime: cabinets, lamps, bookcases, paintings, flower arrangements, old china with impressive pedigrees like Wedgwood — many of them inherited from her mother. Oil portraits of my two youngest sisters hung on the wall. The rest of us had to make do with photos: there were dozens of Mum's children and our families.

Mum greeted me with a wan smile.

I bent to kiss her forehead. 'Not so good, huh?'

'It's all right for me, I don't have to run around after anyone else,' she said. Running around after other people had been her lot.

'Am I first?" I asked.

She frowned. 'First?'

'You know, for your birthday weekend.'

'Oh yes,' she said. 'It's going to be lovely, isn't it?'

Her eyes closed and I tiptoed away to put the kettle on. I'd had enough back pain of my own to know how it could knock the chatter out of you.

I returned with a tray of tea just as the doorbell rang.

'I wonder who that is,' Mum said, opening her eyes. 'I'm not expecting visitors.'

One by one, my sisters arrived with greetings and pillows and bags of food. That night we slept in our childhood combinations. Growing up in our family had been done in pairs. Although the four oldest came pell-mell, an invisible line separated Matt and Liz (the big ones) from me and Rose (the little ones). Just as Mum bundled Rose off to school, the Catholic Church rang to say they had a batch of orphans from Hong Kong who needed good homes. Apparently Dad said, 'Let's take two.' Mum's response to this has not survived. By the time two-and-a-half-year-old Chun Ying (our Ginny) got off the plane clutching a plastic purse, Mum was six months pregnant with Kate, and the final twosome was in place.

As we lay in bed on Saturday morning, Rose told me I'd called out in my sleep. I was surprised. I'd had a nightmare that I was buried alive in a spot so remote I'd never be found. But when I'd tried to cry for help, the black earth had smothered and silenced me.

It rained all weekend. Mum was too sick to go anywhere. The rich food and overheated rooms sapped our energy. The damask gold and aqua wallpaper closed in. It had originally been a bold choice by Mum to offset the sea-green carpet and curtains in their Wadestown house. Ever practical, she'd chosen it again for the Newtown one: it matched the furniture and she couldn't find another she preferred. Somehow its swirling floral pattern symbolised her relationship with Dad across both houses, much of it under a cloud of illness that stopped him in his prime and turned her into his carer.

Up close, over two days, we saw the extent of Mum's confusion that she'd managed to conceal when we simply popped in. If she came across us in a room, she greeted us as if we'd just arrived. She muddled her medication, asked stock questions over and over again, lost track of the conversation, opened *Live Bodies* at the same page every time.

Later, I asked Rose what she remembered about that weekend. 'You were cross,' she said. Our family aren't yellers and screamers. We don't usually slam doors or throw things; we rarely even raise our voices. What we do is get brisk and tight-lipped. We get cross.

Rose was right. I'd wanted to be at the beach. Swing through the sand dunes with a bottle of wine and watch the sun go down. Smell the salt in the air. Feel the surf scour my skin. We'd had family holidays at Waikanae since we were tots — the sight of Kāpiti Island still gives me goose bumps — although eventually Mum got tired of entertaining hordes of Wellingtonians within arm's-length of her hospitality, and insisted on holidaying further afield.

Now we couldn't leave her on her own. We took it in turns to escape into the town belt behind Colville Street. Up there it was cool and quiet where below there was nothing but heat and clamour. The pine needles were slippery underfoot; grey slivers of harbour glinted through the spindly tree trunks. My racing heart slowed as I hauled each breath over the rock in my chest. I wanted to hide forever, free from the ties and obligations of family. I wasn't cross any more, I was desolate. Something was wrong with our mother.

CHAPTER THREE

———

BABIES

ONCE MUM'S WELL-BEING was on our radar, we realised her whole life had to be monitored. The strain was quick to show. Four Wellington sisters. Four opinions about Mum's competence, the help she needed, how best to respond. A dodgy water pipe burst in her bathroom, damaging the walls and flooding the hall. Just as Rose saw off the final tradesman, another pipe burst. The insurance company said they wouldn't pay out if it happened a third time, which meant we'd have to replace all the plumbing.

Then Mum told Ginny she had two cracked vertebrae and wanted to wear a corset like the one that had fixed her mother's bad back. Ginny took her to the orthotic centre only to find that Mum had cancelled the appointment without telling her and it was weeks until another was available.

Ginny and Kate still had young children. Rose and I worried it wasn't safe, or fair, for Mum to babysit them as they sometimes asked her to do. This caused tension — and sadness. We'd had Mum to help us: their kids needed a grandma too. Matt, home for Christmas, tried to organise a family meeting. Rose refused to come. I got cross, then made up with her over coffee, forgetting it was my 24th wedding anniversary and falling out with Pat instead.

Emails became our morse code, the only way to keep Mum's six children in Wellington, Hastings and South East Asia in the loop. Independently, Ginny and I started saving them, she with her secretarial eye, me with my writerly one. Over the next four years we stored several thousand on the subject of our mother. Some were a cryptic line or two, others ran to pages: stoic, distressed, funny, practical, angry, exhausted. They acted as both safety valve and barometer, not only of Mum's well-being but also our own. On a good month there might be half a dozen; on a bad month 40 or more. The medium wasn't perfect. Emails tended to document the crises and fade out during easier times. They were better for dealing with practical concerns than emotional ones. A flippant response, a loaded silence, a missed message could threaten our stretched alliance. But consensus mattered, even if Matt would have liked us to be more decisive and sometimes bristled at his sisters' surveillance.

'Told Mum she didn't need to make shortbread for Hastings as well as 300 mince pies!' Ginny emailed after she'd helped her pack her bag for a reunion of Dad's family in the New Year. Once upon a time, Mum's mince pie claim would have been modest. Now she couldn't make a dozen without help. 'I wonder if Matt is liaising with her at all re time they're going, what to bring — foodwise etc.,' Ginny added. 'Should I interfere and give him a call?'

Liz, who was organising the reunion, had booked out a motel to accommodate the out-of-town guests. Away from the familiarity of home, we got a glimpse of what Des had noticed about Mum on their South Island trip. Every time she came out of her bedroom in her tiny unit, her eyes flicked left and right, weighing up which way to go. Every time she needed the bathroom, she had to ask where it was.

As Pat walked along the driveway one morning, Mum called

out a greeting from her front door. She was wearing her dressing gown and brushing her teeth, he told me in astonishment. He'd never seen his mother-in-law without her face on, let alone in her nightwear with foamy lips.

On a hot Hawke's Bay afternoon, 50 Desmond descendants and their progeny gathered at Liz and Dave's for lunch. We were just one branch of the family tree planted on New Zealand soil by Ellen Burke and John Desmond. John was an Irish private who immigrated in November 1846 with the 65th British Regiment, dubbed 'the 'Hickety Pips' by Māori. It's more likely he built roads than fought in the New Zealand wars. But by his late thirties he'd been discharged from the army as medically unfit, and he died a few years later, leaving Ellen and eight sons.

Poor health dogged many of Dad's forebears, as it dogged him. His grandfather Joseph Desmond, a hansom cab-owner in Wellington, was reputedly a long-time invalid. His father Harold, a bookkeeper, died of pneumonia at 36, shortly before the advent of penicillin. Dad was 10, the oldest of four children, with an overdeveloped sense of responsibility and underdeveloped airways that caused chronic asthma.

His mother Elizabeth May Doherty was also unwell as she struggled to raise her family on a widow's pension. It was only the largesse of a bachelor uncle that got Dad to medical school, where he met Mum. It seems Elizabeth was wary of the girl from the Roxburgh gentry who stole her first-born's heart. But she died a week before their wedding, giving her future daughter-in-law little time to win her over.

Guests of honour at the Hastings reunion were Dad's younger brothers, Joe and Phil, so like my lean, well-spoken father that it hurt. Their sister Kathleen, a Sister of Compassion, had died in her fifties.

If my uncles and aunties, who'd known Mum for half a century, noticed any change in her, they didn't say. Nor did we confide in them. It would have felt disloyal; we hardly knew what to make

of the change ourselves. From the outside Mum looked older —
just like everyone else. As I chopped tomatoes into a salad, she
hovered at the kitchen door, stylish in a crisp blouse and linen
trousers with a dark brown belt. She seemed dazed by the bustle
and clatter where once she'd have been in the thick of things. A
child rushed past and just about upended her. I was relieved to
see someone take her arm. Next time I saw her, she was parked
in a deck chair on the lawn, devoting her attention to one of my
cousins.

That night Mum's teenage grandchildren had a session in the
motel bar. Channelling the cheek — and drinking habits — of the
Irish, they charged their beers to Mum's room. When the sizeable
tab came to light, they high-fived her about her big night and said
she should invite them to her next party. They thought they were
hilarious. So did she. She footed the bill.

AFTER THE REUNION, Pat, Liz and I took Mum to Pourerere
Beach where Liz and Dave owned a log cabin nestled in the only
decent stand of trees on the eroded hillside. Despite our bird's-
eye view of the curved bay and pounding surf, Mum thought she
was back at Waikanae, the setting of so many family holidays.
She was too wobbly to walk on the sand, too disoriented to make
a cup of tea. Every morning she packed her bags to go home.

One day Liz and I brought up her memory loss. Mum admitted
she was worried but thought it had only been a problem for a
few weeks. She hated the idea of being a bother, she said. We
reassured her it was her turn to be looked after. It was a relief to
say it out loud. There was lots of laughing.

Liz kept Mum while I went back to help my Wellington sisters
organise more support for her. Mum had flurries of agitation
followed by long calm spells, Liz emailed. 'It's actually been

lovely having her here and great for the kids to have time with her, and they are great with her.' But Mum fretted that Matt would drive her red Honda Concerto while she was away; she'd become possessive about the car she'd once have gladly lent to any of us. To settle her, we posted her car keys to Hastings where their arrival had the opposite effect. Mum got out the phone book, rang the bus company and made a list of bus times home. 'All under her own steam, which viewed one way is very positive,' Liz said. 'Yesterday she told me she was on this week's Pregnancy Help roster — cunning plan to get back to Wellington, eh?'

The cunning plan turned out to be true. Although Mum was too frail to lug nappies and layettes, buggies and bassinettes to women all over town for Pregnancy Help as she'd done for 30 years, she still manned the community agency's helpline, Kate discovered after Mum's return. 'Had 7 calls written down to prove it! Though I don't know what she'll do with them? (Apparently it's 24-hour cover, but Mum said you'd be very unlucky to get one in the middle of the night!)'

Mum was a founding member of Pregnancy Help, set up during the heated abortion debates of the 1970s. As a Catholic, she believed in the sanctity of life but, unlike Dad, she had little stomach for the hard-line Society for the Protection of the Unborn Child with its strident acronym SPUC.

Pregnancy Help eschewed politics in favour of practical support for women who wanted to keep their babies. Mum never lacked for material comfort but she did know the desperation an unplanned pregnancy might induce. One afternoon, as we sat at her table, I asked her what her own births had been like. The reserved mother of old would have brushed me off. This new one was more frank.

'Yours was the worst,' she said, although that seems questionable: she'd almost died of a post-partum haemorrhage after Kate was born in Wellington. But it was the horror of the maternity ward at Dunedin Hospital she recalled, and I wondered if her first four births, each 14 months apart, had fused into a single nightmare.

'Nobody understood. The pain was terrible.' She covered her face. The 'dragons' at the hospital told her to pull herself together and left her to labour alone in conditions that would be considered barbaric these days; she thought they relished seeing the doctor's wife pulled down a peg or two. Dad — who'd delivered other women's babies in his two years as a GP at the Roxburgh Hydro camp, and was a joyful witness at my son Jackson's birth — waited outside like any expectant father of the 1950s.

I asked Mum how she felt afterwards.

'More dead than alive.' Her voice was barely a whisper. 'If I hadn't had Grandma to help' — she meant her mother — 'I'd have drowned the lot of you. Or I'd have drowned myself.' Her words brought a rush of tears to my eyes, but also a softening around my heart for her predicament — and ours.

Four babies in three and a half years. The Pill was not far away but it wouldn't have helped: Catholicism forbad artificial birth control. I was baby number three. At six months, I refused to eat and was dispatched to Grandma's to be fattened up. This story had always made me feel special. But when I asked Mum about it, she said she didn't have time to spoon-feed a reluctant eater because she was pregnant again. It was the first time anyone had acknowledged the family crisis behind my banishment: Mum's depleted energy; Rose's superior claim in the womb; my unconscious protest that may have caused me to clamp my lips shut.

Whatever the wrench at being separated from Mum for six weeks, Grandma kick-started my appetite by offering me tiny morsels on a salt spoon, I've been told. She was known as Dolly because she was so petite, Des said, but I remember a stately woman with an ample bosom and good legs, her snow-white hair pulled into a bun, her scratchy chin the price of a kiss. When I was three, she took me again. By then we'd moved to Wellington. As

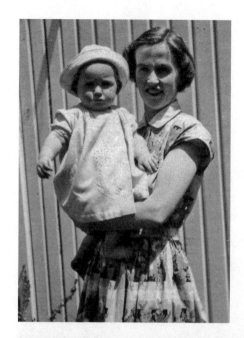

left
Mum embarking on motherhood with Matt, Roxburgh Hydro camp, 1953.

———

below
Our family soon after Mum and Dad moved to Wellington in 1957 with four children under four. From left: Matt, Grandma, Rose, Mum, Liz, Dad, me.

———

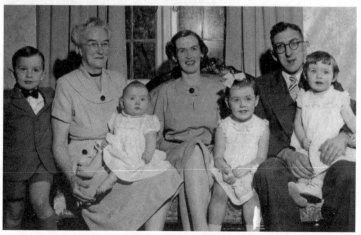

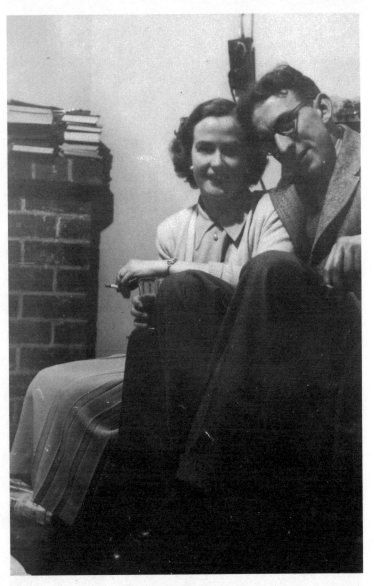

Mum and Dad, footloose and
in love in Dunedin during their
student days, late 1940s.

the two of us were flying to Roxburgh, she fell at Dunedin airport and broke her arm. She kept me anyway, to be her helpmate, thus cementing our bond.

Before this torrent of babies, there's a black and white photo of Mum and Dad. It's a formal occasion: he's in a bow tie, she's in gloves to the elbow and a gown with a complicated neckline. Their heads are almost touching. Half-smiles light both their faces — as if he's just told her she's beautiful, and she knows it's true.

Another photo, around the same time. They sit side by side; behind them is an ugly socket on a bare wall, next to them a stack of books on a mantelpiece. It looks like a student flat or Dad's room in a Dunedin boarding house when he was a med student. His head tilts towards Mum's; her arm rests on his thigh. Thick-rimmed glasses give him an intellectual air. She's demure in a buttoned-up blouse — until you see the glass in one hand and the cigarette in the other. That's when it hits you there was a time before us. A time when they were footloose, worldly; most of all, equal.

Fast-forward to their fortieth wedding anniversary. We threw a surprise party: we didn't want Mum fretting about food and guest lists and whether it would be too much for Dad. He made a short speech (she didn't), then wrapped one arm around her and pressed her cheek against his with his other hand. In the photo, they're beaming. He couldn't be holding her tighter if he tried.

I offer these images as snapshots of my parents' affection from one end of their long marriage to the other. In between times, things sometimes got tricky, as they do. Dad loved Mum and he loved us but he followed his church's teachings without question. Mum, a good Catholic wife, knew the deal and handled the consequences. There was no one to complain to. Which may explain why, for three decades, she'd supported other women who found themselves pregnant, overwhelmed and trapped up or down a heap of steps.

CHAPTER FOUR

PORTFOLIOS

I PHONED THE manager of a new homecare agency and found myself in tears about Mum. Food, exercise and company were our main concerns, I said. She seemed to be losing confidence and withdrawing; she admitted she found it easier talking to people on the phone rather than face-to-face. And her weight, already pitiful, had fallen to 42.5 kilograms, less than seven stone. There was also a problem with her big house. I asked the manager about other living options.

'Why do you want to move her?' she asked. 'A change like that could affect her psychological state, you know.'

I *did* know: removing a single pill from Mum's medicine tray sent her into a tizz. I also knew the advantages of 'ageing in place'. As press secretary to the Minister for Senior Citizens, I wrote speeches advocating it. But until now I'd never considered the place in question might be Colville Street: up a hill, with 12 rooms, a double garage, a huge attic, exploding water pipes, three external doors and slippery wooden steps down to the garden.

I felt let down by Mum. She'd promised she'd know when it was time to move, and I'd believed her. Now she was trapped. It was too late to go, too hard to stay.

The manager suggested that a carer could come in every day to prepare Mum's lunch or evening meal and make sure she ate it. We called a family meeting. Mum wouldn't hear of a stranger taking over her kitchen but she reluctantly agreed to two hours' help twice a week.

I imagined finding someone closer in age to Mum who'd share her interest in gardening and books, or someone younger who'd take her for walks and make her laugh. Someone who wasn't us. To allay her fears about how she'd keep this person occupied (she hated the word 'carer'), we came up with a list of jobs more befitting a cleaner than a companion: weeding, changing the sheets and smoke alarms, cleaning the oven and silver, sweeping the garage, replacing light bulbs. In a letter to the manager, Mum insisted on putting 'helping me with' in front of each task to show who was boss. She ended the letter, 'I enjoyed meeting you last weekend and am so grateful for your help.'

This was not true. The first carer, Lynn, did nothing to allay Mum's fears. A cheerful chatterbox in her early forties, she arrived wearing a black trouser suit, a white hat that looked like she was off to the races, and crystal drop earrings. Mum referred to her as 'that woman' and complained that all she did was sit around talking and drinking tea.

It was hard to know if these objections related to Lynn in particular or the concept of care in general. Occasionally, one of us would pop in to try and gauge the vibe when she was there. But if we were going to pop in, we might as well be there ourselves. And popping in changed the vibe. I muttered to Liz about putting in a hidden camera.

'Do we really want to know how Mum spends her days?' Liz said.

It was a thought too sad to consider.

After each visit by Lynn, there'd be anger and tears and threats from Mum to ring the agency and cancel the arrangement. From Yangon, Matt emailed Mum in solidarity about his own home help: 'My Lynn is called Nay Chi Linn and she's starting to get to me. She keeps moving things to where she wants them — the cutlery, the spare plastic bags, and the rice-cooker. I move them back while she's watching and she says, "Sorry Sayar" — every day. She checks the rubbish to see if I ate all my dinner.'

We reduced Lynn to one shift a week until Mum got used to the intrusion. It was hardly worth the trouble. Every time I saw Mum, she was adamant she could manage by herself. The only line that got through to her was when I blurted in desperation, 'Mum, *you* might not need help but *we* do.' At this, her shoulders slumped and her protests trailed away. The defeated mother was worse than the stroppy one. After I left, I couldn't stop crying.

Lynn added to our logistical headaches. In spite of our emails, we kept tripping over one another. Mum, alone at Colville Street headquarters, was unable to pass on a message, let alone run the whole operation. She ordered a winter's supply of firewood. Rose arranged for her son's friend to stack it in Mum's garage. But when the load was dumped across her footpath, Mum rang me in a panic. She'd forgotten the friend was coming, and I didn't know he was. I spent an hour finding someone else to stack the wood. By the time the friend arrived, it was done. Everyone was cross.

The homecare agency suggested a communication book. Anyone who spent time with Mum could write down what she'd eaten, where she'd gone, whether she'd taken her pills, what follow-up was needed. As well as its practical uses, it would remind Mum who'd been to see her and how she filled her days.

We bought a sturdy book and put it by the phone in the dining room. 'I forgot to write in the book — but would have needed a new book if I'd remembered,' Matt emailed cryptically on a brief visit home. The original had disappeared. A replacement vanished just as fast. The message was clear. Strangers were bad enough; Mum had no intention of allowing the details of her life to be pored over like a tacky tabloid.

To minimise duplication, we carved Mum's life up into portfolios like government departments. I was minister of health, Rose housing, Ginny transport and commerce, Kate internal affairs, Matt foreign affairs and finance, Liz attorney general and state services. Meanwhile, Mum retained her position as our increasingly erratic head of state. In a typical week, every minister was stretched to capacity. As well as our rostered visits and portfolio responsibilities, there were emails, phone calls and family meetings. If Mum's role as matriarch was to keep us connected, she was succeeding beautifully.

THE WELLINGTON HOSPITAL geriatrician was a charming man in his mid-fifties who ushered Mum into his office with a bow. Within minutes she was calling him by his first name and they were laughing like old friends. After a physical examination, he gave her a mental aptitude test that included asking her to remember three things. Five minutes later Mum — who forgot I'd been to see her after five seconds — was able to recall all three.

The geriatrician took his time studying the report of Mum's CT brain scan. Then he fixed her with his warm, intense eyes and told her she had cerebrovascular disease caused by years of high blood pressure.

'Is it dementia?' I asked.

'No.' He raised his eyebrows at Mum as if to say, *Daughters: drama queens.*

Mum raised her eyebrows back.

He turned to her, cutting me out. The disease was affecting her balance and memory, he said, but not her intellect. There was no reason she couldn't drive short distances but he advised against going anywhere new. Stress would make things worse: illness, change, medication. Especially medication. The biggest culprits were Mum's sleeping pills and the Panadeine she took for back pain. She should cut out the latter straight away and wean herself off the former as soon as possible. He'd see her again in two months.

Mum nodded, as if these instructions were reasonable. They weren't. She'd started taking sleeping pills in her mid-forties when Dad got sick. Like many of her generation, she never stopped. She did try. The bottle of sky-blue Triazolam was full of bits: she'd take half when she went to bed and another nibble if she woke before morning.

I was 16 when Dad had his first seizure without warning in the middle of the night. It was so severe that he nearly died and was hospitalised for weeks. Gradually life returned to some sort of normal. Everyone prayed it was a one-off. The following year, Mum and Dad went to Europe, leaving me and Rose in charge of Ginny, 11, and Kate, 8. Before Mum left, she filled the freezer with pre-cooked meals and stashed a fat purse of banknotes in the cupboard above the fridge. Both Rose and I recall Mum saying that the money was to bring them home if anything happened, although on reflection this seems improbable. Perhaps we've reinforced each other's false memory over the years and it was for minor emergencies.

Dad had seizures while they were away, more seizures when they returned. His GP told Mum they'd gradually get worse and one would probably kill him, she confided in Liz. No wonder she hated the violent, unpredictable visitor that felled her husband and shattered her sense of order and beauty. Her dread was infectious, and soon our house was filled with fear. Convinced I heard Dad fall in the shower one morning, I flung open the door, to be confronted by him upright and naked. 'Sorry, false alarm,' I muttered, averting my eyes. The embarrassment was all mine: my father was never prudish about his own body.

Anti-convulsants gradually tamed Dad's *grand mals* into *petit* ones. But the cocktail of Dilantin and other drugs made him drowsy and dizzy, and affected his balance and concentration. To try to reduce the side-effects, he meddled with the doses, increasing the potential for more seizures. He cut down to part-time work at his pathology laboratory and gave up all his good causes except St Vincent de Paul and Medical Aid Abroad.

Mum's life changed dramatically too. The husband who'd never been there needed a driver to go out. The patriarch who'd made decisions for them both couldn't think his way to the end of a sentence. The success story who'd defined her place in the world withdrew from it. For a while, she drank gin in the afternoon. Together they went to see a psychologist. After a couple of sessions, they declared it mumbo-jumbo, though Mum later told Liz they stopped going because Dad couldn't stop crying. No one talked about the effect on us kids.

Occasionally a big one struck. After cracking his head open as he fell, Dad was sent to Australia for a CT scan; such scanners were not yet available in New Zealand. Ten years after his first seizure, the machine that would one day show the damage to Mum's brain revealed a slow-growing, inoperable tumour in Dad's. Radiation helped. The fits subsided, Dad began driving (badly) again and a small hiatus opened up for both my parents.

But the tumour continued its slow march and on Easter Sunday 1994, my father died at the age of 67. Three hours earlier, Mum had taken a sleeping pill. When Liz woke her with the news, she got out of bed and shook off her grogginess to face her first day as Fred Desmond's widow. Since then, the small blue pills had helped her get through the long nights alone. No, I was not about to wrestle them off her now.

After the geriatrician visit, I stopped at Colville Street for a glass of wine. We were both feeling light-hearted. Mum was finally under the care of an expert in older people's health, and the news wasn't as bad as I'd feared. She could keep driving. With help, she could stay at Colville Street. We'd replace the Panadeine with Panadol, worry about the sleeping pills later. Best of all, she didn't have dementia. I'd seen a Canadian documentary about a woman with Alzheimer's disease who packed her suitcases with bananas and didn't recognise her daughter. Mum wasn't going to end up like that.

She confessed she was self-conscious about her memory loss. 'It's like my brain's a little person.' She grinned. 'I might give it a name.'

'Cybil?' I suggested for no good reason.

'No, I think of it as male.'

'Not Fred, is it?' I asked.

She laughed, refusing to confirm or deny.

ON A SATURDAY morning in late summer, I found Mum sitting straight-backed in a red leather armchair in the study that overlooked the street, drawn there by the early sun. Her white hair, usually puffed up in a perm, was flat against the sides of her head, making her look tinier and more vulnerable than ever. She greeted me through swollen lips that she'd smothered with cream meant for her sun-damaged hands. She 'was a bit of a mess, and needed lots of hugs,' Ginny had emailed after discovering the mix-up.

Half the small room was taken up by Dad's roll-top desk with its leather inlay, secret drawers and cubby holes. When I was growing up, he'd always had a place to do his important work where he couldn't be disturbed. It had never occurred to me — or Mum either, I suspect — that she might like a room of her own too. Her important work was to look after us and she had the whole house for that. Although she left us largely to our own devices, her décor, her industry, her order, her smells formed the comforting backdrop to our lives. On the rare occasion she took to bed with a migraine or a bad dose of flu, we crept about, subdued and out of sorts, as if someone had turned all the lights off.

These days Mum stacked her bills and letters in a manila folder on the roll-top desk as if she hoped its gravitas would help her deal with them. Above the desk hung a large Dali painting of Christ on the cross suspended in a dark sky above a lit-up bay. I avoided looking at it. Not because of the crucifixion — such scenes peppered my childhood — but because the towering, tortured Christ felt too much like my father, the tiny fishermen caught in his omnipotent gaze too much like me.

When I asked Mum what she was doing, she told me she had to sit upright for half an hour before taking her weekly bone density pill. I got the pill and a glass of water and said the half-hour was up. I didn't have the heart to tell her (again) that the upright instruction was to aid digestion *after* taking the pill. Nor to ask why on earth it would be before.

After making her tea and toast, I coaxed her into her clothes and off to a jazz concert a few blocks away. At the entrance to Carrara Park, she clutched my arm and took small, scared steps along a path lined with a bright animal mural. Some distance from the band, I unfolded deck chairs and put my jacket over her knees. Couples sprawled on the grass. A shirtless boy in a trilby hat danced alone to the languid sounds. A woman chased a toddler. I broke the news to Mum that we'd have a baby of our own soon: Megan was pregnant. Mum's pleasure at the prospect of her first great-grandchild calmed me, reeling from the unexpected news I'd be a grandmother at 50.

The outing brought colour to Mum's cheeks. But by the time I got her home, her back was bothering her again. I asked if she'd like me to massage it. In the past she'd have turned me down and dealt with her pain in private. Now she gave me a grateful smile. As she bent forward in her chair, her sleeve slipped up to reveal a bandage on her mottled arm. The wound had appeared from nowhere and needed regular dressing by her GP. With no fat to plump up skin as thin as tissue paper, healing came hard.

I ran my fingers down the knots and bumps along her misshapen spine. No wonder she was convinced she had cracked vertebrae. I asked her what would make the biggest difference to her quality of life.

'Being able to walk properly,' she said. 'And not being so tired.' I was surprised. For me, her memory loss overshadowed everything.

'How tired *are* you?' I asked.

'I'm tired all the time.'

'Do you think you're depressed?'

'No.' A deep sigh rose from her chest. 'But I could be if I gave in to it.'

CHAPTER FIVE

———

WONDERLAND

WHEN DES ANNOUNCED he was coming to stay at short notice, Mum was rattled. 'I'm not good company at the moment,' she told Ginny. 'And what is he going to do for a week?' Visitors had become unwelcome witnesses to her disintegrating world. But she relaxed as her brother fixed things around the house, took her on outings, gave her space and didn't pry.

They seemed so alike, given how their lives had diverged. After Mum went to boarding school, except for school holidays they never lived in the same town again. While she became a wife and mother, he joined the Christian Brothers' teaching order and moved to Australia. Twenty years later, he left the order to marry Chris, an ex-nun, a thrilling act of subversion in my then-teenage eyes. Despite the ripples it must have caused at home and in the church, Mum and Dad both went to the wedding. After that, Des settled in Adelaide and only came back occasionally — as if he were in exile, self-imposed or otherwise.

Grateful for the reprieve of our uncle's visit, the rest of us scarpered, asking him to share his thoughts about Mum when he got home. In a long email, he said she was much frailer than when he'd taken her to the South Island, but agreed she should stay at Colville Street for as long as possible. His reasons were the same as ours: familiarity, exercise, independence, the pleasure she got from her garden, the stress of moving out. He also listed the negatives: not eating, loneliness, the possibility of leaving the stove on or having a serious stroke or fall. He warned us to check her credit card regularly for withdrawals by unscrupulous charities, something that had never occurred to me.

'What you are all doing at this stage is wonderful and there is no doubt in my mind that Rosaleen would not be as well as she is without all the love and care she is receiving from each of you,' he said.

It was good to have his blessing; sometimes letting Mum live alone felt like neglect. But his suggestions that she accept a carer every day and that we ask the geriatrician to spell out the progression of her illness and present her with a list of options for the future — 'It is essential that Rosaleen "owns" the option which she decides upon. She may not like it but [it] is her choice' — seemed as impractical as removing her sleeping pill. I couldn't even get the geriatrician to say there was a problem.

Matt also wanted to put his foot down. Perhaps it was a boy thing or a lack of time spent in the trenches. 'After reading Des's thoughts and being with Mum on Sunday, I'm more convinced that the room for her choices has shrunk further,' he emailed. 'There has to be someone (besides us) regularly in the house. If Mum tells me again she's just eaten a "nice piece of scotch fillet with lovely little new potatoes", I'll scream. And I'm sure her driving days are truly numbered. If you think it will help the decision-making, I will spell this out to Mum very firmly. Problem is with mixed messages — she'll just shut out the firm line, and respond to the vacillating one. I really think her choice this week was Lynn or no hairdresser.'

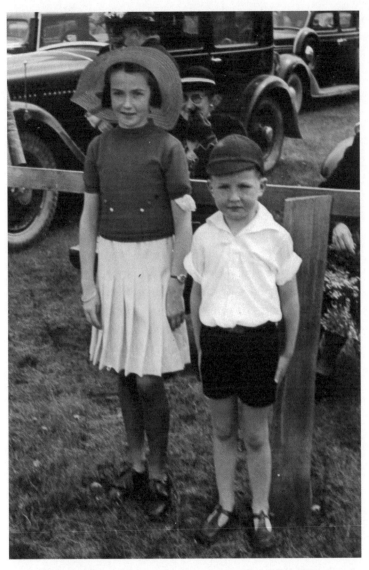

Mum and her brother Des at the Beaumont races in Central Otago, around 1939. Behind them is the family car, a 1936 Chevrolet, and their Aunt Sarah (seated). 'For lunch on a day like this there would be hot soup, hot chicken and vegetables, and dessert to follow,' Des said.

We'd decided it would be safer for Lynn to drive Mum across the city to her weekly hair appointment in Wadestown — and a better use of Lynn's time than re-polishing the silver, the only job Mum would let her do. Except that Mum refused to go with Lynn. Matt thought we should have cancelled the appointment, presumably to teach Mum a lesson. But consequences only work if you can remember that Y happens when you do X. Mum couldn't remember the stand-off, let alone the fallout. Her hair appointment was the highlight of her week. It seemed unfair to make her miss it when the following week she'd just refuse to go with Lynn again.

While he was home, Matt also resisted being tied to the daily roster we'd set up. I understood that it took the spontaneity out of seeing Mum and made it feel like a duty. That's because it *was* a duty. I found the roster practical and reassuring. My free time was my free time. When it wasn't my turn to keep an eye on Mum, I knew Rose or Ginny or Kate would be. Which is not to say I didn't sympathise with Matt. Mum's clinginess, repetitive behaviour, denial about her state of mind and resistance to change were driving me crazy too.

LIZ AND I took Mum to see *Since Otar Left,* a movie about three generations of Georgian women who live in the same house. Mum chortled all the way through at the grandmother's scheming to get her own way. Afterwards, we arranged to meet at Colville Street for dinner. I'd bring a salad, I said. Mum pulled out a shopping list for half a dozen hot cross buns, a bag of lemons, some honey. I said I'd pick them up too.

When I arrived, a salad was already sitting on Mum's bench. In the pantry were half a dozen hot cross buns, a bag of lemons, a new jar of honey. When Mum appeared, I demanded to know why she'd asked me to do her shopping if she intended doing it herself. I'd rushed home, picked fresh greens from our garden and made a special trip to the supermarket. More than cross, I stomped around the kitchen, flinging limp leaves out of Mum's salad and replacing them with my own. As I rinsed a knife under the tap, I caught sight of my reflection in the window. Behind me, Mum stood cradling her shoulder with one hand.

Ashamed, I turned around. 'I should go out, come back in and start again,' I said.

'Or just go out.' Mum's face was stony. Beneath her gentle exterior there'd always lurked the sting of a Scorpio. But this coldness was new. Over dinner, she talked to Liz as if I wasn't there. 'I wonder how the doctor feels about Pip *marching* into the surgery with me?' she asked my sister.

'She'll think you're lucky to have someone who cares about you,' Liz said.

Mum's voice rose a notch. 'And what would Dave think if a patient took notes?' Liz's husband Dave was a urologist.

'He'd be pleased they were so on to it.'

Numbly I chewed on a piece of smoked chicken, Mum's default offering to visitors because it required no cooking. Poor Liz, who came to stay every few weeks, had begun to dread the sight of it. Mum had always told me she appreciated me taking her to appointments, keeping track of her ailments and medications. Now she ranted at Liz about being checked up on and losing her independence.

When I couldn't stand it any longer, I told Mum it wasn't my fault, her memory loss was to blame, and felt a grim satisfaction to see the fight go out of her. Even then, it didn't occur to me that she hadn't deliberately doubled up on the salad and the shopping. She'd have simply come across the list again and headed off to the supermarket like the conscientious hostess she was. My actions must have seemed as irrational to her as hers had to me.

What strikes me now is how capable she was, given how little recall she had of the immediate past. How hard her brain must have been working to appear normal. How spirited her defence when she was caught out. In some ways, her competence was her downfall. She could still fool me into thinking I was dealing with the old, rational mother whose life was well organised and executed. Strangers didn't stand a chance. If we left her to fend for herself, as she pleaded, she presented so well to the outside world that no one realised anything was wrong. After a meeting or appointment, she'd have no idea where she'd been or what she'd said or what she was meant to do next. Then it would fall on us to unscramble the mess.

If Dad had been alive, he'd have borne the brunt of her confusion — taken her to the doctor, paid the bills, filled the cupboards, protected her from nosey parkers. We'd have just thought she was getting a bit dotty. It didn't seem fair. She'd spent 20 years caring for him after he got sick, not to mention all the running around before that. But when it was her turn to be looked after, there was no dedicated minder in the wings.

After the salad debacle, Liz and I agreed we had to step back, that Mum was feeling smothered. 'We can't make her better,' Liz said. 'A lot of what we're doing is for us.'

I thought about the effort we'd been putting into getting Mum to eat. The result after six months was that her weight had dropped another kilo. So when Mum rang to tell me she'd phoned the electrician because her jug and toaster weren't working, I didn't go round to check. I'd get tied up for an hour. I was no handywoman. It would be like saying I didn't believe her.

She looked sheepish when I called in later. 'You know that button on the jug you have to push down,' she said. As for the toaster, she didn't know why it had been playing up. It worked fine for the electrician. He was such a nice man that she'd made him a cup of tea. In fact, he'd only just left.

I wondered if the nice electrician would add the tea-drinking time to his call-out fee. Mum was so vulnerable that anyone could dupe her. She'd just spent a fortune on two crowns for her teeth that the dentist said she needed. There was no way to get a second opinion when she only told us afterwards. Stacks of charity begging letters lay around the house; as Des had warned, Mum seemed to have got herself onto the books of every fundraiser in the country. Whenever he was home, Matt made it his personal mission to destroy them but the reply-paid envelopes were usually gone.

Anyway, it was Mum's money to spend however she wanted. We were lucky that day-to-day she was pretty frugal. She never bought new clothes or splashed out on expensive wine. For another three or four dollars, she could get something decent, I'd grumble as I pulled a bottle of cheap plonk out of her fridge. She didn't care: she only drank a thimbleful. It was me who hankered for something with a bit more class.

A FEW NIGHTS after the salad incident, Mum rang. The conversation went something like this:

'Hi, Pip, how's your flu?'

'I'm fine, thanks, Mum. I don't have the flu, luckily.'

'I was going to pop round with a cake.'

In the past this would have been something homemade and delicious but I knew better than to get excited. 'That's a lovely thought but I'm OK. Really.'

'How are Pat and the kids?'

'They're fine too, thank heavens.'

'I hope they don't have your flu.'

'Nope, we're all good as gold.'

'Oh well, I'd better let you go. Wrap up warm and stay home. You don't want to spread bugs.'

Next morning, she appeared at the back door with a chocolate cake from the supermarket. 'You're still very pale,' she said. 'How's your flu today?'

Looking back, I should have welcomed the cake as a gesture of concern, perhaps even a peace offering. I should have applauded her remembering overnight that I was sick, even if it was a figment of her imagination. I should have savoured the glimpse of the old mother who was always dropping off a fish pie or chicken casserole to feed my family. Instead I just felt weary, as brain-fogged as her, trapped in the circular logic of Wonderland:

'But I don't want to go among mad people,' Alice remarked.

'Oh, you can't help that,' said the Cat: 'We're all mad here. I'm mad. You're mad.'

'How do you know I'm mad?' said Alice.

'You must be,' said the Cat, 'or you wouldn't have come here.'

CHAPTER SIX

CIRCLE THE WAGONS

From: Kate
To: Rose; Ginny; Pip; Matt; Liz
Sent: Wednesday, April 6, 2005 09:23 PM
Subject: Who else!

Hi guys,
Took Mum to Karori cemetery today to say hello to Dad.
Informed her that both Fred & the pope died on April 3rd,
but only one of them [Dad] made Easter Sunday! Had lunch
out after (though she later told Ginny that it was Rose who
took her — I've lost my Brownie points) and she ate well
and seemed good. Despite the fact that she has a sore leg
after falling earlier in the week (?Monday). That only came
out after I questioned her about the antibiotics on the
bench. Apparently she tripped on the utility room doorstep

and gashed her leg. Took herself to the GP the next day and is on regular dressings and yet another ACC form! I guess the good thing is that she wants to use her new stick now.

The saga continues . . .

TTFN
Kate

After phoning Mum all day and getting no reply, I called round. She told me she'd been at the doctor's because her leg was still not right. I asked what she'd done with Lynn who was meant to be there. She'd fired her, Mum said. For good. In writing and by phone. It wasn't working and she didn't want her any more.

Worn out by her resistance, I said we'd respect her decision. Then, in a futile bid to lay down consequences of my own, I said I hoped she'd be all right by herself on Lynn's day in future.

Mum tried to look contrite.

When I got home, I rang the homecare agency. The manager said Mum hadn't cancelled the service but she'd reduced it to once a fortnight (which was why Lynn hadn't been with her) and she'd been phoning a lot to complain. We agreed it was time to take a break. As Matt observed, Mum had manipulated me into delivering the knockout punch on her behalf. I could almost hear the glee in Liz's reply: 'Objectively it was a terrific little exercise in self-determination — and personally I'm blaming that movie about Otar!'

EIGHTEEN MONTHS AFTER Des raised the alarm, six months after the geriatrician said Mum had cerebrovascular disease that affected her memory and balance but not her intellect, we were back to square one. Apart from her sore leg, Mum did seem sprightlier: her back pain had inexplicably disappeared and her balance had improved. If anything, this made her more of a menace. Every time we looked, her Honda had another scrape that lined up with the side of her garage. She blamed everyone else: Matt, her grandchildren, rogue trollies in the supermarket carpark. We contacted her insurance company to explain why a third panel-beating claim was on its way, and warned the Honda service centre not to give her a replacement car while hers was being repaired yet again.

For now Mum had won the battle to drive herself to the hairdresser. After one appointment, she told me her brakes had failed on the way home. I asked her what she'd done. She just kept driving and pumping them, she said. Implausible as this sounded, the thought of her careering down steep, windy Wadestown Road was too disturbing to dismiss.

'What about other cars?' I asked.

'I moved over to the outside lane.'

'Why didn't you stop?'

'I didn't have a cell phone and I didn't know AA's number.' She gave me a reproachful look as if this was somehow my fault.

'You could have asked someone to help.'

Mum considered this, then changed tack. 'I'm not a dill. I tried two garages. Both of them said they didn't have mechanics, so I kept going.'

The Honda workshop could find nothing wrong with the brakes but suggested replacing the master cylinder, at a cost of several hundred dollars, to be on the safe side. Then Mum told Matt it was the accelerator that had failed and concocted a different story about how she'd got home. If her testimony became unconvincing, she'd veer off in a new direction. She never backed down or admitted she was wrong. Never. Especially when it came to driving, which she defended as passionately as her right to stay at Colville Street. Mum had ferried Dad around for years after seizures stopped him driving. She'd seen his frustration at being dependent and the burden it placed on both of them. So when a government pamphlet came through the mail with a proposal to abolish the compulsory practical driving test for 80-year-olds, she underlined the relevant paragraphs and left it on the dining room table for all to see.

Soon after, Mum took a wrong turn and ended up on the motorway to Petone, a 30-kilometre round trip. Perhaps she (who could hardly remember the jug button) should get a cell phone with all our numbers stored on it, she suggested to Matt. 'Are you serious?' Liz emailed when she heard. 'Ideally, it's a great idea but practically, **&$#@#!!!'

Safety aside, we were as desperate for Mum to stay behind the wheel as she was. Without the car, she'd be stranded. She'd never caught buses and there was no way she could walk down to the Newtown shops on her stiff legs and swollen ankles.

To check her driving prowess, I got her to pick me up for her next appointment with the geriatrician. She found our house and managed to back into our lane, but I had to direct her to the hospital, which was visible at the end of the street. On the way there her speed was rather erratic but she didn't do anything unpardonable. I gave her a C minus.

After seeing Mum's latest back x-rays, the genial geriatrician sympathised with her pain and agreed she should use anti-inflammatories in short bursts when it got her down, another blow for his drug-free goal. Mum had three compressed vertebrae, osteoporosis and spondylolisthesis, a condition that affected her lower back and made her legs feel weak, he said. If she fell, she'd probably break something. She needed sun every day and the more she walked, the better her balance would be. The stairs at Colville Street were great.

Mum looked smug at this endorsement. She did glide up and down those stairs with ease. But it was almost impossible to get her to walk outside. No sooner would we be through the gate than she'd complain about the wind or the cold, the sun or the pitch of the footpath, and demand to go back. If we made her take a walking stick, she'd swing it beside her like Fred Astaire. Her main exercise was trundling around the supermarket with a smoked chicken and a box of Eskimo pies in the bottom of her trolley, which doubled as a walker.

Not that I could discuss any of this with the geriatrician. After telling Mum she had cerebrovascular disease on her first visit, he never brought up her memory loss again, nor asked how we were coping as a family. Mum sailed through her appointments, giving me no opening to discuss our qualms. If I produced examples of her forgetfulness, she'd get huffy and deny them. He'd side with her; they'd both turn on me. His exclusive patient focus, no doubt admirable in other contexts, fell down when the patient was an unreliable witness to her own life.

Mum's regular GP also avoided her memory loss. Mum insisted she had to go and see her every month, whether she was sick or not. She remade appointments as quickly as I cancelled them and began turning up at the surgery unannounced. I hoped this might convince the GP that there was something wrong with Mum beyond her cuts and bruises.

Meanwhile, Mum kept asking the GP and the geriatrician for more prescriptions until she had enough drugs to cover a national emergency. I begged my siblings to always fill her prescriptions at the same chemist so we had a central record. I was finding it impossible to monitor her drug-taking — especially her sleeping pill — if she kept rushing off and getting more little bottles and tipping them into each other.

Following my plea, Ginny drove Mum's Honda to the nominated chemist and left Mum sitting in the passenger seat while she went in. When Ginny came out, the car had gone. Hoping Mum was the culprit and that she'd head for home, Ginny started walking. As she slogged up the hill, Mum drove past her. When Ginny arrived at Colville Street, Mum opened the door with a smile and said how nice it was to see her.

MUM WAS WORRIED about Matt's next visit. After the last one, she told me, he'd made her stop at the bank on the way to the airport and withdraw $10,000 to pay for his plane ticket back to Myanmar.

'Plane tickets don't cost ten thousand dollars and you never buy them at the airport just before you leave the country,' I said, trying to strangle this train of thought at birth.

She shrugged. 'Oh, well, I don't know. That's what happened.'

When he was home, Matt oversaw Mum's financial affairs, perhaps fuelling her suspicions about his intentions. When he wasn't there, Ginny set up a manila folder for her bills and correspondence so they could go through them together. But Mum accosted us all with the contents of the folder. 'She has told me on a number of occasions that she had to take over the bills when Dad got sick and she had absolutely no idea what to do/ how to go about it,' Rose emailed. 'I wonder if she's been anxious about them for 20 years!!'

Mum was certainly anxious about them now. She hounded the bank for statements and cheque books, the accountant for her tax return, the dentist for receipts. She banked the insurance cheque for food that had spoiled when her freezer mysteriously turned itself off, then swore the cheque hadn't arrived. Her response to direct debit notices for her rates and insurance was to fire off cheques for an equal amount.

'Mum is going to the supermarket and buying I don't know what but managed to go Monday and Tuesday and spend well over $100 each time (I know it's easy to do) but really I wonder,' emailed Ginny. She also found receipts for one large order of wine, then another, although there was no sign of the wine itself.

After a fruitless hunt for Mum's Work and Income client number and the paper trail to show whether her MASS medical alarm was still being funded as part of her disability allowance, Rose had had enough:

From: Rose
To: Kate; Ginny; Pip; Liz
Sent: Wednesday, September 7, 2005 08:11 PM
Subject: Mum, money and MASS

Well sisses,

Personally, I feel quite strongly that this stuff cannot be dealt with 'by the next person who goes into the house'. It is far too complex and thwarted by so many differentials (like no bank statements and Mum's sheer confusion) and I, for one, have no idea what has happened before or with whom or when. Multiple people cannot deal with these matters and they are perhaps better left undealt with or left until 'the' person can check on it — maybe in this instance Matt after 26 Sept?

Before I left the house, there was a phone call from a tree company saying they had received and banked a cheque from Mum for work they had not done. They had only given her a quote for work that could be done in 3 weeks' time! I have followed them up on it and they are to post back to her a cheque for $285 & GST that they had quoted. Thank God for honest folk. He was horrified about the other company's $450 quote for the same job . . . Much room for thought on this one. Mum was so totally and utterly confused by it all that she couldn't even remember who she had been speaking to as soon as she put the phone down. We could not locate the cheque book from which that cheque had been written so there was no chance to check it all out — nor whether one has also been sent to the other company or . . . I think we should leave it there and wait to see if/when their invoice arrives. Though I reckon Mum is not capable of dealing with her bill payments any longer . . .

And nor were her pills taken today.

And two frozen dinners were sitting in her fridge . . .

Lovely note to leave y'all on. This is not at all easy — and I know I am more upset than she is . . .

xxxxxxxxRosexxxxxxxxxxxxx

The kisses on either side of Rose's name looked as if they were propping her up. She and I had power of attorney over Mum's affairs. To invoke it, we only had to fill in a form at the bank. But any suggestion that we look after her personal cheque book ramped up Mum's anxiety even more.

There was a freneticism to her activity, as if she were trying to replicate her busy housewife role of old. Our portfolios buckled under the strain. As government departments discover, people's needs don't fit neatly into separate boxes; they clash and overlap in awkward ways. Sometimes I wondered if it might be easier to be an only child, a single port of call, all-consuming as that would be.

Mum somehow managed to draw the six of us into her web of half-truths and false leads, bewilderment, omissions, vagueness and wild goose chases. Left on her own, she'd ring us one after the other, sometimes several times a day, often with different versions of the same story. We had to be careful not to believe what she told us, especially about each other. Nothing, no matter how convincing, could be taken at face value.

THE CALENDAR THAT hung in Mum's pantry provided growing evidence of her jumbled circuitry. It was an old-fashioned one with big squares, garish flowers and a twee poem for each month. As 2005 unfolded, biro entries in Mum's elegant handwriting made way for multi-coloured capitals in thick felt tip — as if by writing boldly enough, she could sear the information into her brain.

Single words began to fill, and sometimes over-run, the squares: 'LIZ' — 'HONDA' — 'ELECTRICIAN' — 'LUNCH' — 'DRESSING'. As the months went by, the white squares and border vanished beneath names, numbers, question marks, arrows, brackets and asterisks. Entries were crossed out, written over, underlined, boxed, circled. Looking at the calendar was exhausting, trying to make sense of it impossible. If this was the window to Mum's mind, all was not well.

Amidst the muddle were occasional pointers to her old social life. 'Lunch Joan.' 'PH [Pregnancy Help] AGM 7.30 p.m. Anvil House. Clare to pick up.' 'D.O.Gs [Dominican Old Girls] 11.30 Portland Hotel.' Getting her to attend such gatherings was another matter. She'd often cry off outings at the last minute, saying she felt sick or her back hurt. Increasingly she wanted to be with us — and only us.

Mum had never been a joiner. She hated the idea of bowls and housie, and refused to sign up to exercise classes at the Arthritis Society when her joints flared. Throughout her life, she'd always had a few close friends, usually quirky. Her bridesmaid Margaret, a fellow boarder at St Dom's, became an air hostess in the days when it was still glamorous, and went on to crew the King of Jordan's private jet. She had no idea what to do with us kids when she breezed into town in her blue soft-top MGB sports car, but she put a spring in our mother's step.

Jeanette was another doctor's wife with a big brood, but she took time out from her unruly family to produce paintings good enough to sell, and delighted Mum with her irreverent views and mimicry.

Then there was Rosemary, whose non-church-going husband,

three children (only) and paid job were all noteworthy in our circles. It was she who quizzed me about the nun who was persecuting me at primary school when I went to play with her daughter one day. Undone by her kindness, I poured out my woes, then felt like a traitor for confiding in the wrong mother.

When Rosemary dropped me home, she and Mum spoke in low voices. Next day, Mum and Dad took me aside, one of my few childhood memories of having their joint, undivided attention. I think Mum confronted the nun. I know she did when the same thing happened to Rose. Boarding school had left her with a loathing of bullying.

Mum had other friends too: funny, lively women with whom she ignored the housework, talked louder, laughed more. When five o'clock struck, out came the gin and up went the hilarity. But such occasions were rare. They lived all over town or overseas; they might chat on the phone but their usual get-togethers were ladies' lunches and dinner parties with their husbands, which took a week of preparation when it was Mum's turn to be hostess. Day-to-day, she spent her time alone — or rather with us, her children — a product of her class, her generation and her temperament.

Mum got on well with men too. After she and Dad moved to Wadestown, she struck up an unusual friendship with the bearded gardener who came to help maintain their challenging section. Mark trimmed the macrocarpa on the driveway and swung the lawn mower around the grassed terraces while Mum dug and weeded and tended her flowerbeds. When the work was done, they'd sit at the kitchen table drinking tea or gin, yakking about plants and fine food, books and raising kids. After Dad got sick, Mark became even more of a fixture in our house, his offbeat company as vital for Mum as his gardening skills.

I don't know what happened to Mark but by the time Mum began to lose her memory, Margaret and Rosemary had died and Jeanette was looking after a sick husband. The names on Mum's calendar showed there were other people who cared about her. We sometimes wondered why they didn't rally around more or ask us what was going on. On the other hand, we had no idea what she was saying to them and how many offers of help she was turning down.

As with Dad's brothers, we didn't reach out to Mum's friends either. It was hard to know who to trust: people could be clumsy and patronising, and Mum's emotional radar was finely tuned. She'd have been furious — and mortified — if she thought we were talking about her behind her back. In hard times, you circled the wagons and kept your troubles to yourself. That's how she'd coped with Dad's seizures. Outsiders had no idea how deeply his brain tumour rocked our family, the cracks hidden beneath her spotless house and stoicism. Now we followed her lead. What would we have told them anyway? We still didn't know what was wrong ourselves.

CHAPTER SEVEN

DIFFERENT MOTHERS

ON 9 SEPTEMBER 2005 I watched my first grandson come into the world and was awestruck by the tenacity of life on one hand and its fragility on the other. The baby was named after his father Rome, a New Zealand-born Samoan. Megan and the two Romes spent half the week at our house and half at his parents'. When Mum met my new son-in-law, he took a gentle interest in her.

'Your English is very good,' I heard her say after they'd been talking a while.

'Thanks, I've been practising.' His expression was deadpan.

'Where are you from?' she asked. It was clear she visualised coconut palms and white sand.

'Lower Hutt,' he said, referring to Wellington's neighbour.

'And where did you go to school?'

Rome named St Bernard's College, also local. At this, Mum got it into her head that he'd been a boarder at St Bede's College in Christchurch and that his family still lived in Samoa. Whenever she saw him, she'd commiserate about how far away they were.

Such misunderstandings did not enter into Mum's relationship with her great-grandson. We'd sit her in an armchair and prop the baby in her lap with cushions. Her face would light up as she gazed into the dark pools of his eyes and stroked his dimpled fingers with her gnarled ones. 'I love babies,' she'd say.

When I think of Mum now, it is her hands that come to mind. As the rest of her shrank, they seemed to grow bigger. In later years, she was ashamed of the swollen, red knuckles and ropy veins, the age spots, sores and scars, the brittle nails as lined as her face. But to me their twisted beauty spoke of a lifetime of toil and care. They never failed to soften something inside me.

In her younger days, no matter how many pots Mum scrubbed, gardens she dug or shirts she washed, those hands were moisturised and manicured, adorned with her jewelled wedding and engagement rings. Once a strange man took them in his own on the steps of the Basilica Cathedral and told her she had the fingers of a pianist. I was 10, and the compliment felt shockingly intimate and misplaced. It was *me* who played the piano, unthinkable that my mother would pursue such a frivolous, private interest of her own.

Mum's creativity took more practical forms: cooking, sewing, needlework, gardening, flower-arranging, interior decorating, calligraphy. Liz remembers her having a good singing voice — her father was church choirmaster in Roxburgh for 47 years — but I only recall her shyness at having to sing hymns at Mass after Vatican II.

She could paint too, if the Venice scenes in oils she'd done as a young woman were any indication: they were paint-by-numbers but skilful all the same. Des told Liz that Mum gave up painting for us kids — the implication being that she shouldn't have. After that, she confined her artistic talent to daubing gold trim on the plaster curlicues she glued to every wardrobe door at Wadestown Road.

MUM, MEGAN AND I went down to the Chinese Baptist Church in Newtown to cast our votes in the general election. It was Megan's first outing since her baby was born and she seemed as disoriented as her grandmother.

Before we'd set off, Mum had asked me who she should vote for.

'Whoever you think's best,' I said, resisting the urge to launch into a spiel about National's 'Iwi versus Kiwi' racist fearmongering and Labour's last-ditch promise of interest-free student loans that might save her grandchildren from penury. A few minutes later, I was glad of my restraint when she announced she always voted National because her father had. Her roots were thoroughly blue. A photo of National Prime Minister Sid Holland had hung in John Harry Waigth's home office in Roxburgh, and he'd been secretary of the Central Otago branch of the National Party when he died. Nothing I said could compete with the pull of history.

A week later, I sat in my office at Parliament waiting to see if I still had my press secretary job. Labour had won by a nose but National refused to concede defeat until special votes were counted. To pass the time, I flicked through a pile of community sector magazines. One from Alzheimers New Zealand caught my eye. Inside I read that a dementia epidemic was looming and that vascular dementia caused by high blood pressure was the second most common kind.

Before I lost my nerve I dialled the phone number provided for the Wellington branch. When the manager, Carol, answered, I blurted out my fears about Mum.

Carol was kind and blunt. Everything I described about Mum

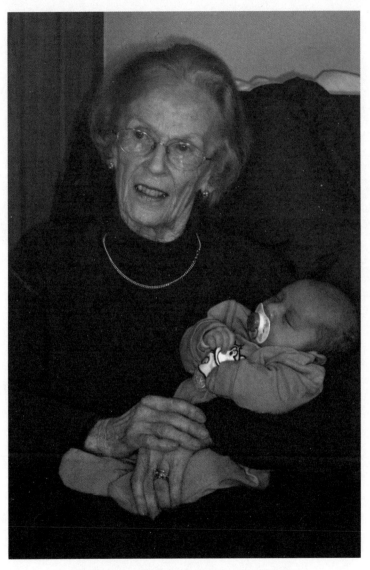

Mum loved to hold her first great-grandchild, Rome,
born in September 2005. The twisted beauty of her
arthritic hands spoke of a lifetime of toil and care.

— cutting herself off from friends, losing interest in activities, immediately forgetting people had phoned or called in, presenting well during health assessments as her survival instincts came into play — fitted her experience of dementia, she said.

Questions tumbled out of me, my grief tempered with relief that the monster might finally have a name. Carol told me the symptoms of Alzheimer's disease and vascular dementia were similar and often overlapped, but the latter was usually a 'step' decline as mini-strokes deprived parts of the brain of oxygen, while the former was a more gradual 'hill' decline as brain tissue shrank. People with dementia had good days and bad days just like everybody else, she said. Mum might stabilise for a while but she'd continue to deteriorate. How fast was impossible to predict.

I asked if it was safe for Mum to live alone. Carol said people with dementia rarely hurt themselves by forgetting to turn off the stove or crashing the car. The biggest risk was of wandering and getting lost. Not for Mum, I thought, whose aversion to walking suddenly turned into an asset.

With every other medical condition, you'd let a person choose their course of action, Carol said. Dementia was different. Mum was never likely to say it wasn't safe for her to drive or live alone. Any hint of change would only make her try harder to hold onto what was familiar. Her ability to reason was affected so there was no point arguing with her. The right time for Mum to move was when the family couldn't cope any more.

She followed with a string of warnings that reminded me why we felt so paralysed. You could leave it too late to change someone's living situation, she said. Mum's ability to adapt would only decline. But it was very hard to take someone with dementia into your own home. Even those with the best intentions found it terribly frustrating. And if we opted for supported accommodation, we should choose carefully. A lot of retirement villages didn't have facilities as the disease progressed, and people had to move out again.

When I emailed my siblings with Carol's informal diagnosis, no one was surprised. 'I accept that Mum has dementia,' Rose replied. 'I think I have known it for some time but I, too, am glad it has now been given a name.'

However, the hospital geriatrician remained non-committal. In a private phone call — I knew better than to bring the matter up in front of Mum — he said lots of people with memory loss like Mum's didn't develop dementia, and if she did have it, it was just in the early stages. He said we needed to proceed gently before making changes to Mum's life and recommended a psycho-geriatric test.

Ginny took Mum to her next hospital appointment. 'He asked how Mum was and of course she said "Fine",' she emailed afterwards. 'I said it was hard work for four of us coping with her memory loss and other behavioural obsessions. He says, "Just relax!" I said, "It's all very well for you to say that, you don't have to live with it!!" He says, "Does Mum look worried?" And there she is sitting with a big grin on her face looking very serene (at that stage my blood pressure was probably higher than Mum's). End of conversation as far as he was concerned.'

The geriatrician might have thought he was sparing Mum — and us — by making light of the situation. But his flippancy was as unhelpful as his advice at Mum's first visit that cerebral vascular disease was affecting her balance and memory but not her intellect. At the time I took his word for it. I'd grown up in a medical household believing doctors were all-knowing and powerful. Dad's long illness and my own intractable back pain had dented this certainty but my childhood reverence of the profession was hard to shake.

These days I'm more sceptical. While I was writing this book, I looked up 'intellect' in *The Oxford English Dictionary* and found it meant 'mental powers; faculty of reasoning and understanding objectively'. It was hard to see how the geriatrician could have thought Mum's mental powers and ability to reason were unaffected by her memory loss — so I decided to ask him. But when I googled his name, I discovered he'd died just two years after Mum, at the age of 64. It came as a shock: he'd seemed so robust, so in charge, so sure of himself. My conviction that doctors are our healers took another hit.

ROSE RAISED THE possibility of Mum moving in with her and her husband Mike. Their Miramar house was ideal in many ways, with flat access and a stand-alone room on the back lawn that could be converted into a bedsit. Mum would have regular company and better care, and the chaos of Colville Street would disappear. But so would all the things that filled Mum's day: small domestic tasks laid down by years of patterning, unlikely to survive the move.

We called a family meeting. It had become impossible to include Mum in these pow-wows but she was the only subject on the agenda. As usual Ginny took notes and sent out the minutes. The atmosphere was tense. Rose wanted us to actively encourage Mum to move in with her. Matt and Ginny were in favour, but the rest of us had reservations.

As Liz emailed afterwards to Rose, 'I hope you know that I think it's wonderfully generous and that we would be behind you every step — financially and otherwise. Unfortunately I suspect that it will be a trial and error situation with no real way of knowing whether Mum'd settle into it or not.'

And what if she didn't settle? I knew how difficult Mum could be if she felt she was being railroaded. I worried she might blame Rose — or me — for making her leave Colville Street. I worried about Rose's expectations of the rest of us, and the conditions she might set if Mum couldn't be left alone, as seemed likely. I worried about Mum feeling abandoned if she got too much for Rose and had to leave. Beneath my fears ran a deep vein of guilt.

That my heart wasn't as big as my little sister's. That I wasn't up to bringing Mum home to live with me.

Nevertheless, if Mum had agreed to move in with Rose — or with Liz, who'd made a similar offer — I think we'd have backed the idea. But Mum didn't agree. She told Liz she'd be stuck there. She wanted to stay where she was. She wanted nothing to change. And so we dithered, trying to accept the ever-widening gap between the life Mum yearned for and the one we could deliver.

It was getting harder to leave her on her own. When we organised another girls' weekend at Waikanae, we took her with us — although I longed to be free of her. Not just her haphazard mind but her knotty back and joints; her anorexic weight; her low blood pressure (after years of high) that could lead to a fall; the infected callous under one foot; the sores on top of the other; the precancerous growths on her face and hands; the endless doctors' and specialist visits; the bureaucratic tangle around her entitlements.

On the first day at Rose's beach house, Mum was sweetly bewildered. By the second, she was restless and pacing, packing her bag, pestering to leave. Conversations about her future were impossible. On the way home, she asked, 'Aren't we going on holiday?' and complained she hadn't seen Liz, who'd just driven off, for weeks.

Our weekend together reminded me that each of us was dealing with a different mother. These mothers might sometimes coincide or intersect but they'd never merge. That had always been the case, of course. Dementia just heightened the stakes.

My mother was prickly and critical but also had moments of deep confiding. Rose's seemed kinder, perhaps in response to Rose's patient, unwavering love. Liz's was soothed by her eldest daughter's calm authority. Kate's accepted her youngest daughter's matter-of-fact nursing style.

Ginny's was difficult in a different way to mine. She'd started accusing Ginny of stealing things. Ridiculous things: her placemats, her walking stick, her TV remote control, her salt and pepper shakers. When Ginny arrived in our family as a fearful toddler, Mum had slowly won her over by tempting her with fried eggs and letting her play in the pot cupboard. I prayed she wouldn't undo all their years of mutual devotion now.

After a three-month absence, Matt described his mother in an email:

From: Matt
To: Rose; Ginny; Pip; Kate; Liz
Sent: Tuesday, October 4, 2005 14:37 PM
Subject: Re: whanau meeting

I've spent a lot of time with Mum the past 5 days after none for 3 months. Yes she forgets a lot more a lot quicker. The big changes I notice are:

That she can now get quite obsessive. Maybe this is thru having to fix on something even harder to get it together. The obsessive behaviour that worries me most is the hours she spends in her cheque book.

That she can be 'manipulative'. Maybe this is just forgetting from one minute to the next what she just did or said . . . my hunch though is that she's rather conscious of what she's doing . . . almost being naughty after all these years of being good.

That she is more anxious and less trusting. Maybe there is a part of her that's getting ready for a fight. That my Wgtn sisters are less 'forgiving' of her little cock-ups and games. Even if this is simply exhaustion, I don't think it is a bad thing. I suspect it will become more and more appropriate to relate to her almost as a child. I will find this very hard — to acknowledge that she's seldom the savvy, gracious, self-sacrificing Mum I've always known.

However . . . she continues to get done what's necessary to get through the days. There are also some very strong survival instincts in there. I've seen her cook (I'm sure her appetite has improved), make her bed, have a bath, light the fire, do the shopping . . . all with efficiency and aplomb. It will be good, Pip, to have a look at what her living options might be. I'm not sure she needs to move yet, but I am sure that when the time comes it will be us who make the call.

Matt

'I'm not sure that I have become less forgiving — of her,' Rose replied. 'I just know that more and more I want to spend my time with Mum having the best possible relationship — not fixing up the world that's constantly 'collapsing' around her. xx A very sad Rose.'

WHEN I DECIDED to tell this story, I found comfort in the existence of all these mothers. If there were so many versions, it was impossible to betray the one, true Rosaleen Waigth. No matter how deep I dug, her essence would remain intact, unknowable. What I was doing was wrestling with the mother in my head.

Back then, it was hard not to envy those with easier relationships with Mum. Somehow my mother and I always seemed to end up at loggerheads, often over her health. As we did on the wet November afternoon when a psychiatrist, nurse and registrar filled Mum's stuffy lounge with their black coats, brollies and briefcases. No one had told us the psycho-geriatric assessment would require a team of three experts. I left Mum in their clutches while I made coffee. When I returned with a tray, the psychiatrist asked her if she had any concerns about her memory loss.

'No,' she said. She sat in her chair by the fire like a sullen child, her scrawny arms folded, her mouth set in a grim line. She might not have known exactly who these people were but when it came to sensing danger, she was an expert.

The psychiatrist turned to me with an enquiring look. I felt my cheeks flush. Surely he didn't expect me to contradict Mum in front of his team. That's why we'd called him in, to get an independent opinion, so we could stop being the bad guys. I muttered something about being worried about her.

'What for?' Mum said sharply, and I retreated into silence.

My heart sank as Mum answered the usual questions about her age and address and the day of the week, drew the correct time on a clock face and made a perfect copy of a diagram. I hoped the psychiatrist realised these tests were a waste of time for her. The only time she faltered was when he gave her three words and asked her to repeat them a minute later and 15 minutes after that. By the second time, I'd forgotten one of the words myself.

He asked about her driving. 'Warning signs are things like little dings going in and out of the garage.'

'We've had a few of those,' I ventured.

Mum put on her haughtiest voice. 'You know who's done them, don't you? One. Of. My. Daughters.' She might as well have pointed at me.

I suppressed an urge to laugh. Overall, though, the visit was depressing. The psychiatrist said there was no test to determine a person's level of dementia or the right time for them to leave their home. It was up to us to judge Mum's safety. In fact, it was up to us to do everything, it seemed, including cover the cost of his two recommendations: a $500 private driving assessment for Mum and an exorbitant cognitive enhancer called Aricept that wouldn't cure her but might boost her memory and awareness for a while. Unfortunately one of its main side-effects was nausea, the last thing she needed when she was already off her food.

After the team had gone, Mum and I huddled at the end of her dining table, wrung out, soft with each other. She mentioned she needed 'supervision' when I think she meant to say 'support', a slip-up so astute my eyes pricked with tears. Then, as if to rectify the error, she said, 'I'll know when I can't live here any more, but I don't think I'm ready to be shipped out yet.'

Afraid of losing hard-won ground, I plunged into the unspeakable. 'At some stage, it's going to come down to three choices, Mum,' I said. Fear flickered in her eyes but I ploughed on. 'Someone can come and live with you.'

'*Hmmph*,' she snorted. 'A boarder. That would be the end of *me*.'

'Or you can come and live with one of us.'

'*Hmmph*. That would be the end of *you*.'

I swallowed hard. 'Or you can go into some sort of supported living.' I avoided words like 'rest home' and 'care' but both of us knew what I meant.

When she finally spoke, it was in a whisper. 'I hope I die before that happens.'

CHAPTER EIGHT

SILVER WEDDINGS

MUM FELL AGAIN. She only confessed when Kate rang in the middle of the day and found her in bed. She had no idea how it had happened but her gardening shoes lying willy-nilly on the back step, the gash in the back of her head and the bloody blouse in the laundry bucket provided some clues. Her head wound required two stitches and Mum was bruised and in shock. She needed help with everything, including getting dressed. We added our husbands and kids to the twice-daily roster.

Pain increased Mum's confusion. So did new drugs to combat the pain: antibiotics in case of infection; Voltaren for inflammation; Losec for nausea. Concerned she was overdosing on Panadol, we hid the box of 500 given to her by the GP, and scoured the house for hidden supplies.

Every Saturday, Mum and I sorted her pills into seven plastic drawers, one for each day of the week, divided into morning and night — the same system Dad had used when he was sick. But the new pills threw her. She took some, left others, muddled the doses. With trepidation, we took up someone's suggestion to trial blister packs put together by the chemist: less room for error and random consumption. But Mum had no idea what to do with the packs and fretted about the seven empty plastic drawers.

Four days before Christmas she rang before breakfast and began reading me the report she'd received from the psychiatrist. It must have arrived in the mail the day before; I wondered what she'd done with it in the intervening hours. The report referred to her in the third person. It said Mrs Desmond had early dementia that would get worse; that she should consider not driving and might not be covered by insurance if she continued without an assessment; and that her GP could get the Land Transport Safety Authority to seize her licence if she was deemed to be unsafe. Mum was crying now. Why did the report say her family were increasingly concerned about her safety living alone, she wept? And why did she need the phone number for Alzheimers New Zealand?

I was as dismayed as Mum. Surely, I thought, the psychiatrist could have predicted her reaction at seeing the dementia diagnosis in print; her obsession over every (death) sentence; her despair at the prospect of losing her licence. He knew she lived alone. Surely he'd have realised she needed support when she read the report, which was why I'd asked him to send it to me, not her.

Mum veered between anger and anguish. She rang several times a day accusing me of dobbing her in, threatening to drown herself in the bath if she couldn't drive. If I'd had the psychiatrist's personal phone number, I'd have given it to her.

On Christmas Eve I went round to check on her. Darkness was falling but her front door was unlocked. I let myself in. There was no sign of life: I could have burgled the place — or worse. I called out. A minute later, Mum came up the stairs looking flustered.

She breathed nicotine and peppermints over me in a reluctant hug. She'd always been a secret smoker, hiding cigarettes under Dad's fedora in the hall cupboard and other odd places. I didn't call her on it; for years I'd been one myself. Clandestine smoking had the double advantage of preserving her dignity and limiting her intake.

Mum took me through to the dining room, picked up a piece of paper off the oval table, the nerve centre of her world, and handed it to me. I braced myself for another diatribe. But the paper was a list of her 18 grandchildren written in her elegant hand. She wanted to give them all some money for Christmas, she said. This was the mother of old speaking, the one who always remembered their birthdays and what they were up to. She'd put $20 in an envelope for each of them, she continued, but now she couldn't find the envelopes. 'I think I must have posted them. Yes, that's what I did. Have your three got theirs?'

Even I didn't know the addresses of the boys' flats. Megan's words came to mind: *Talking to Grandma is like playing Pick-a-Path.* I chose the diplomatic path. Maybe the money was on its way, I said.

'Well, I definitely got it out of the bank,' Mum said. 'I remember all the notes. Yes, I must have posted them.'

'Hmmm,' I said, not wishing to escalate hostilities.

She gave me a sharp look. 'Now you're humouring me.'

'Perhaps you're thinking about what you used to do,' I suggested.

'Or maybe I remember what I wanted to happen.' There it was again, that disarming flash of insight.

'It doesn't matter, they don't expect anything,' I said.

She seemed to accept this. As I was congratulating myself on the ceasefire, she reached behind the pink and white cyclamen on the table and held up a small plastic bag. On it was stamped *Bank of New Zealand.* It was empty. Her eyes danced with delight. 'Now do you believe me?'

I laughed and sent the troops a text message: 'Know anythng abt Mum giving the kids money for Xmas?'

Beep, beep: I've got it safely at my house (Ginny).

Beep, beep: Ginny's got it at her house (Kate).

Beep, beep: No idea (Rose).

If nothing else, our call-and-response skills had become finely honed.

AS 2005 DREW to a close, Pat and I inherited our family's wedding shield. We'd first presented it to Mum and Dad in honour of their silver anniversary. Liz and Dave were next to achieve the 25-year milestone; Rose and Mike would make it within the year. Des had told me our forebears were known as 'the much-marrying Waigths'. We were becoming the long-marrying Desmonds.

Pat was rightly proud of our staying power. Mired in a menopausal funk, I didn't feel worthy of any pedestal, marital or otherwise. However, I managed a short speech during which I told the four-generation clan gathered at Ginny and Gabe's that the main thing I'd learned was to never come between a man and his lawns. At this Mum threw back her head and laughed. We'd only just convinced her not to mow her own lawn any more, fearing she'd sever the cord of the electric mower or worse, her foot.

At 50, I felt less sure of who I was than when Pat and I had exchanged our marriage vows in the tiny church within spitting distance of Mum and Dad's Wadestown house. After the ceremony, Mum hosted a dinner for our mismatched families. The next day, she helped cook the wedding supper for 150 guests, including seven different sorts of pavlovas: a miscalculation as it turned out because everyone wanted to try them all. Even in those days she was no pushover. When a group of patched Black Power members from my gang connections commandeered two platters of freshly caught crayfish, she strode over to their table, took one back and gave them a lecture about manners.

Mum never interfered in our relationships or choices of partner. But I knew she liked Pat from the moment the afro'd son of a freezing worker swept me off my feet at university in the mid-1970s. It took me a long time to realise I wasn't rebelling as much as replicating her courtship with Dad, another boy from the wrong side of the tracks. On his first visit to the Roxburgh homestead, Dad is said to have surprised Mum's father by helping himself to a second beer with unseemly haste before whisking Mum away in a rental car.

My lanky boyfriend had a motorbike. When he turned up at Wadestown Road one night, Mum ignored the helmets under his arm and spied a new pair of white socks between his frayed jeans and grubby sneakers. 'Why, Pat, you're looking very neat about the feet,' she said.

I left them watching TV while I got ready to be whisked away myself. Later, Pat said a Cockney boy had come onscreen hawking his goods in a London market. 'Untouched by 'uman 'ands, me muvva-in-law made 'em!' the boy cried.

Pat chuckled into his substantial beard.

'What did he say, Pat? I didn't quite catch that,' Mum asked, though there was nothing wrong with her hearing.

'It wasn't very funny,' Pat mumbled.

'Well, you're certainly laughing a lot,' she said with a smile that let him know he should never underestimate her.

Mum only got properly cross with him once, he told me: when she discovered I was planning to hitchhike the 400 miles from Wellington to Auckland alone, as I often did in my twenties. 'I don't know why you let her,' she scolded him. Pat shrugged, as powerless to stop his headstrong girlfriend as she was.

After we graduated, Pat and I went separate ways: he on his OE, me to share the lives of gang women. While Dad saw my involvement with the women as a kind of missionary work that aligned with his strong sense of social justice, Mum was less enthusiastic about the danger her daughter might be putting herself in. She coped by not talking about it and feeding anyone I brought home. I took her forbearance for granted and wished she'd be more outspoken.

'You think too much,' she'd say as I railed against yet another injustice against women or Māori or the poor. In my youthful arrogance, I thought she didn't think enough. After a Sunday newspaper published my first feature about the new phenomenon of out-of-school care, I was thrilled when Mum sent me flowers, but dejected when she showed no interest in the article. Pat's mother, on the other hand, spent an hour debating every point with me over the phone.

By our mid-twenties Pat and I had tested our independence and moved in together. Dismayed that we were living 'in sin', Dad forbad Mum (and Ginny and Kate, who still lived at home) from crossing our threshold. Mum didn't openly defy his ban but slipped us supplies whenever we went to see them. 'There's only one thing I ask,' she said. 'Don't get pregnant.' I failed her in that as well but it was too late for scolding and she got on with loving her first grandchild, then two more.

With a baby on the way, Pat and I decided to get married to keep the family peace. Afterwards, Mum helped me paint the den of iniquity and assemble the things I'd need for motherhood. Left to my own devices, Megan might well have slept in a drawer. And while Mum made it clear she wouldn't provide childcare while we went out to work, she was always there as back-up. Six times over, for each of her children — until she got dementia.

In spite of living close by, Mum never intruded on my life or arrived at our house without a reason, usually to give me something. When I did manage to entice her inside, she'd be onto the dishes, folding the washing, peeling the spuds. It sounds churlish, I know, but sometimes I wished she'd just plonk herself

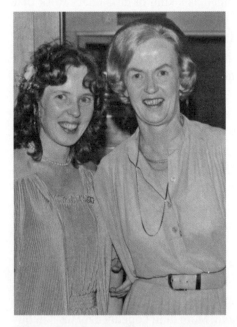

left
Mother and bride,
19 December 1980.

———

below
Our family on
my wedding day.
Standing, from
left: Liz, Matt,
Rose, Ginny, me,
Pat, Kate. Sitting:
Mum and Dad.

———

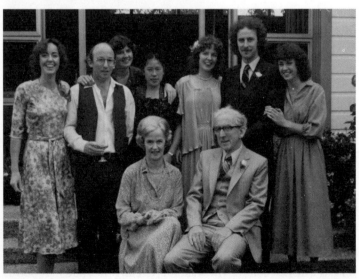

down, tell me to *put the kettle on, I'm gasping*, and settle in for a natter, like my mother-in-law did.

Now she was calling in 50 years of favours. 'It really struck me this time how Mum uses us like an anchor rope,' Liz emailed after coming down to stay with her while the rest of us took a summer holiday. 'The endless questioning felt like constantly checking where the shoreline was and that the rope was secure — without that she must feel like she's adrift in unknown waters. That thought helped me to hold it together, anyway, though I did feel a little nutty myself after a few days! I have to say that I wonder how long she can last at Colville St — really, she is pretty extreme, but you all know that.'

Indeed. Which was why, when the builder said he was ready to start renovating our kitchen and bathroom, Pat and I decided to move in with friends while the work was being done. When Rose heard, she emailed asking if we'd considered staying with Mum. I knew she'd recently found Mum lying on the couch in her nightie, unfed, at one in the afternoon, but her question sent me into a frenzy.

Of course I'd considered moving in with Mum. We needed a roof; she needed care and company. The truth was I couldn't face it. I'd just quit my job at Parliament and was about to go back to university. I'd finally carved out the space to write about my years with gang women in the seventies. Apart from two workshops a week, I'd be at home working on my book. For that I needed 'a piece of quiet' as one of my kids used to say. Not Mum pestering me all day, muddled and agitated, sucking the air from my lungs and turning my brain to mush.

When I was a baby I'd been too much for my mother. Now my mother was too much for me.

CHAPTER NINE

—

DRIVING TEST

WE STUMPED UP $500 for Mum's driving assessment, wondering what people who didn't have that sort of money were meant to do. Reading the report still makes my heart ache. Mum did the off-road test first. In spite of the torn rotator cuff that limited movement in her right shoulder, she passed the physical and coordination sections. The standard written road test took her a bit longer than it should have, but she scored 19 out of 25, just below normal. Rating her own driving, she gave herself a 'good' or higher in every category except night-time vision. She was upbeat about her ability to keep driving and said her family was supportive, adding the comment, 'They like me to be independent'.

A computer-generated driving test followed. Mum had to sit behind a wheel and steer a car on a screen in front of her. She scored dismally trying to stay centred on the winding road and racked up numerous scrapes and crashes reminiscent of the real-life dings in her Honda. Then she had to choose between three foot pedals — accelerator, brake and horn — in line with instructions that flashed onto the screen. It seemed tough: Mum had never used a computer. And whoever heard of a horn pedal? In all categories, she scored an unconditional fail.

The assessor advised her to seriously consider retiring from driving. Mum received this feedback 'with devastation', he noted in his report, the only reference to her feelings. Knowing how much was at stake, she insisted on doing the on-road test. If courage was the criterion, she'd have passed with distinction.

There were four people in the car: Mum and an instructor in front, the assessor and Matt in the back. We'd made him take her, on the grounds that he wouldn't be around afterwards to cop the flak. Asked to choose a route, Mum opted to drive to Rose's in Miramar. According to the report, she demonstrated adequate control of the car most of the time. But she stopped at a roundabout when she had right of way, selected the wrong lane and had to turn left instead of right, braked heavily to let in merging traffic, almost hit a truck, pulled over for an ambulance going the other way, then forgot her destination and drove home.

'The issue is not one of Mrs Desmond's physical driving but clearly impaired cognitive function,' the assessor wrote. He recommended immediate retirement from driving and that her licence be formally revoked.

Mum didn't blame Matt for losing her licence: she blamed me. In spite of our pleas, the driving report, like the psychiatric one, was posted directly to Colville Street, wrongly addressed to 'Rosalind Desmond'. Again it was written in the third person. Again Mum read it alone. The second paragraph began, 'Pip Desmond (daughter) referred Mrs Desmond for a full Driving Assessment.' It might as well have said 'Pip Desmond (daughter) turned off mother's life support.' By the time Liz had the nous to remove the incriminating page, the words were etched into Mum's normally fickle memory.

She rang over and over again, slamming down the phone when I answered, then redialling. When I stopped taking her calls, she left distraught messages on my answerphone.

I WENT ROUND to try and make my peace. Colville Street was only a 10-minute walk from our house, past renovated bungalows, a council housing project, run-down cottages with tatty net curtains and armchairs spilling their stuffing on verandahs. Just past my sons' old kindergarten, I snapped a sprig of lavender off a bush, crushed its purple flower between my fingers and inhaled the lemony scent like smelling salts.

On Constable Street, traffic streamed in both directions. I turned right and dragged my feet past Hiropi Street where I'd lived in my first gang house. Right again into Coromandel Street, and the grade got steeper, the dwellings bigger, although the burnt-out shell of a reputed tinnie house brought down the tone. Mum had never walked these streets, even when she could. She was an incongruous Newtown resident, blue-rinsed and well-heeled, a rural South Island girl not used to jostling with a hundred cultures. Although that's not fair either. For two decades, she attended Mass and helped out at St Anne's, the local Catholic church, where most of the congregation was Pasifika and migrant. And every year she and Dad had their neighbours over for drinks, which is more than I do with mine.

Colville Street was a quiet cul-de-sac on the edge of the town belt, an area real estate agents liked to call 'Newtown Heights'. As I got to Mum's gate, I stepped aside for her elderly neighbour who was riding towards me on an old-fashioned bicycle. Mum said the neighbour wobbled all the way into the city. Once she'd shown Mum where she hid her bike behind a pillar at the Town Hall while she did her shopping.

No sooner had I opened the door than Mum advanced on me down the hallway, wild-eyed and screeching. 'You told the doctor. You went behind my back. Your behaviour is despicable.' With each new accusation, she wagged her bony finger at me. I tried to defend myself but she raged without pity, as if a storm had taken up residence inside her.

She was too frail to sustain it for long. The colour drained from her face and she started shaking. 'I have to sit down,' she said. 'My back hurts.'

I helped her into the red leather chair in the study and kissed her forehead.

'I won't cry,' she said, covering her face.

'Go on, have a bawl.' I was fighting back tears myself.

'No. Crying never changed anything.' Then, her fierceness dissolving, 'I'll cry when I go to bed tonight.'

I waited till she was quiet, then fled, leaving her to her demons. At home, I took to my bed. My throat was too raw to speak. It didn't matter; there were no words for how I felt. For three days I wept. Mum would always blame me for losing her licence. It was the dementia, but it was also what she thought about me: that I caused trouble; that I went behind her back; that I named things better left unsaid. My grief felt irrational and overwhelming. There was nothing I could do to make her better. Even worse, there was nothing I could do to make her see me.

I sought the help of a counsellor. For a long time my all-powerful father stalked my psyche. Bit by bit Mum emerged from the shadows. When I slept at all, my nights were full of dreams. Of babies, abandoned and drowning. Of an abundance of food I, and they, could never eat. Of hair-raising car rides in which I was rarely the driver. In some, Mum was a distant, enigmatic figure. Once she hovered above me like a raven, trying to peck out my eyes. The dreams felt more real than reality. I drifted through my waking hours, grieving not only for the mother I was losing but also for the one who went missing when I was a baby.

At a psychology workshop, I learned that courage sits below neutral on the energy scale: it can see us through a crisis but ultimately it depletes us. To thrive, we need positive emotions like love and joy in our lives. Gritting our teeth, soldiering on, doesn't work indefinitely.

AFTER THROWING OUT the spoiled food in Mum's fridge one Saturday morning and sorting her pills into the weekly drawers, I went through to the lounge. Usually she helped with these tasks, but she'd retired in a huff as soon as I arrived. Blaming me for losing her licence had become a destructive, looping thought pattern that seemed impossible to intercept. There was no one to help me distract her: Pat and my boys were at rugby; Megan was pregnant again and living out in Stokes Valley with Rome's parents; my sisters were already in overload.

Mum looked up from a *North & South* magazine, her stare dull and dismissive. I felt as graceless as she was, unable to rise above my own bad humour. 'I'm off now,' I said.

She saw me to the door. As I climbed the few steps to the street and unlatched the gate, she called in a small voice, 'Thank you. I don't know what I'd do without you.'

I turned around but stayed where I was. 'I don't know what you'd do without me either.'

'I'd be in a rest home if I didn't have you girls.'

I was fed up. 'Yes, you would.'

'I do appreciate what you do, you know.'

I went back to where she stood on the porch. 'I know it's hard, Mum, but you've got to stop fighting us. We're doing our best to keep you at home, but you're making it impossible by being so angry all the time.'

'I'm not angry.'

'Yes, you are.'

'I'm not angry with *you*,' she tried.

'You're especially angry with me.'

'Oh!' She became conspiratorial. 'Because you told the doctor about—'

'Your memory?' I was past pussy-footing around. 'Yes. But that's not why you failed your licence. You did a test. It's not safe for you to drive.'

'I don't suppose I can sit it again?'

I shook my head.

'It's just that I hate being a burden.'

'When you brought Grandma up from Roxburgh to live with you, did you think, here comes the burden?'

'Of course not.'

'There you go. That's what families do, Mum, they look after each other. You have to let us in. You can't manage by yourself any more.'

She seemed to shrink in front of me. 'Just give me some time. And please. Don't put me in a home.'

I pulled her close and felt her heart pound under her ribcage like a small trapped bird. She barely reached my nose, although once she'd been several inches taller than me. How had it come to this? How had our mother's fate ended up in our hands?

My mind went back to a conversation we'd had in the same spot a decade earlier. For quarter of a century, Mum had been Dad's carer. By the end, her emotional well had run dry. When the hospice sent him home against her wishes, and it seemed that he might live forever, she called in a favour from the Sisters of Compassion, his sister Kath's religious order. Dad died in their hospital in Island Bay a few weeks later.

'I promise I'll never put you in care,' I'd said, as we comforted each other on that bright summer's morning. Beside us, the white and purple agapanthus blooms along the fence line shimmered in the sunlight.

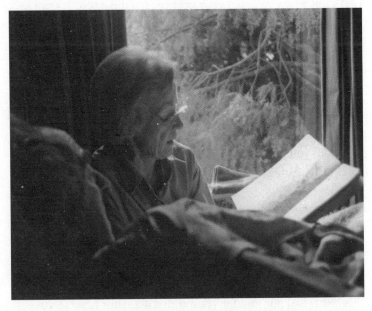

Mum reads to Dad in his final weeks at Colville
Street, early 1994. She cared for him in his illness for
more than half of their four-decade marriage.

———

She turned to face me and gripped my arms. 'Take that back!'

I laughed. 'Don't worry, Mum, you'll be easy to look after. We'll all be squabbling to have you.' I'd meant it. It was in her nature to go quietly, no fuss or bother, just as she'd lived her life. And if she did need looking after for a while, she'd be the perfect house guest: considerate, adaptable, self-effacing.

Her eyes bored into mine. 'You don't know that, Pip. Anything could happen. Now take it back.'

To please her, I took it back.

Now I wondered which mother we should heed. Both wanted to be independent but the early one put her children's needs centre-stage while the current one fixated on her own. This was not a simple case of right and wrong. While the former was undoubtedly easier to be around, I had a grudging respect for the new one fighting for her life. If the meek and mild mother had stamped her foot more, we might not be in this mess. After Dad died, Mum confided that her GP had not properly monitored her high blood pressure and that Dad had been distracted. A doctor in the house can be a dangerous thing, like a plumber who leaves their own tap to drip. Besides, he was the sick one; there was only room for one person in that circle. So Mum put his needs before hers.

When she told me this, I was furious with my father, with her GP, with the lethal power of the medical profession. And I was dismayed at my mother's passivity, her willingness to kow-tow to authority, especially men's. It took months to convince her to leave the GP, such was her loyalty and unwillingness to cause offence. When her blood pressure was finally under control, we thought Mum had been lucky to avoid a stroke. What we didn't know was that mini-strokes known as TIAs, or transient ischemic attacks, imperceptible on their own, were gradually cutting off the blood supply to her brain, stealing her balance, her memory — and, yes, her intellect.

CHAPTER TEN

THERAPEUTIC FIBBING

MUM REFUSED TO relinquish her driver's licence. Her car keys sat in the brass dish on her hall table and her red Honda stayed in the garage. When we suspected she was still going for the odd spin in it, we took the keys. In the course of a single morning, she phoned to say she needed them back to get the car serviced, then because she wanted something out of the boot, a third time because a friend had told her she should turn the motor over regularly. Her brain may have been addled but it was inventive.

Working on the principle of out of sight, out of mind, we asked Mum to lend the car to Megan. The grandmother of old would have gone out of her way to help a struggling grandchild, especially a pregnant one about to have two children 14 months apart, an experience Mum knew well. But she refused to let the car go. In fact there was little sign of the mother on the porch who'd said how much she appreciated our help, admitted she was scared and asked for time to come to terms with leaving Colville Street.

'So what's the point of having those conversations?' I e-wailed my siblings. 'And if we don't have them, what's the point of anything?'

Liz came up with a plan. She flew to Wellington, told Mum her own car had broken down and asked to borrow Mum's to get home. A few days later, Liz rang Mum to say Dave had offered to sell the Honda on her behalf and give her the cash. To our surprise, Mum agreed. She trusted Dave with vehicles: he was always tinkering around with one sporty number or another. She also liked the idea of getting money, a growing obsession. But the real reason became clear when she told Rose that Dave was going to find her 'another little car that she could just have there in her garage'.

Without wheels, Mum was stranded. No matter how much we visited and took her out, there were too many hours alone, and not enough brain power to fill them. At the end of a long afternoon at Colville Street, Ginny sent an exasperated email: 'Mum does not need any more front door keys — I have sorted them out today — she has six. Remote controls for garage doors hanging on hooks inside garage by the internal access door. TV is working, always has been, always will be — she is pressing the wrong buttons! I do not have her long-handled duster!'

After Mum's latest fall, we'd gone back to the homecare agency. But she hated outside care as much as the first time and was on to her fourth carer in as many months. Her night-time phone calls escalated. I imagined her wandering through the empty, silent rooms in her big house as darkness closed in.

Resolving her living situation took on new urgency when Rose and Mike said they were thinking of selling their house in Miramar if Mum didn't move in with them. To help us make a decision, we compiled a list of aged-care facilities on Mum's side of town, and requested a formal needs assessment.

After visiting Mum at Colville Street, the needs assessor phoned to say she didn't appear to be unsafe, thanks to our daily visits and Liz's regular overnight stays. Her biggest concern was Mum's weight. She suggested fruit juice supplements instead of the milk-based ones that Mum detested. Increasing a person's calories could increase their appetite, she said. She agreed it was a good idea to get a feel for rest homes but said what we were looking for now might not be what we needed when the time came. She obviously didn't think the time had come yet.

Just as I hung up, the phone rang again. The acting manager of the homecare agency sounded shaken. Mum was ringing two or three times a day to complain about the service, request invoices and timesheets, change the arrangements and allege no one ever returned her calls.

I told the woman that we'd support the latest carer, the best one yet, but we had enough battles of our own with Mum and the agency needed to deal with her phone calls. Out of curiosity, I asked if they received calls from other clients; it was hard to believe Mum was the only crotchety old lady on their books. No, she said. Most didn't have the agency's phone number; their children organised the service. Could I take the number off Mum?

Any sympathy I had for her evaporated. Mum had written the agency's number in her pop-up index pad, a record of everyone she'd regularly phoned over 30 years, I explained. If I crossed it out, she'd be furious. Besides, she was quite capable of looking it up again in the phone book. *One more call to you, one less to us*, I thought.

The manager said she'd go round and talk to Mum. I hoped this was a good idea.

A few days later, Mum claimed her wedding rings had gone missing during the carer's shift. Rose and the carer scoured the house, to no avail. Later, Rose remembered that Mum often soaked the rings in a glass of dishwashing liquid. Sure enough, there they were on the windowsill above the kitchen sink. The carer understandably resigned. Without consulting us, the agency replaced her with two new carers on the grounds they needed 'as robust a system as possible in place'. Only the system wasn't robust for Mum. The carers came on different days, doubling her potential for confusion and indignation. The agency also said that if Mum's phone calls didn't stop, they'd have to consider charging her for the time they spent dealing with them.

RATHER THAN ENDURE another harangue from Mum, I bundled her into the car and took her to watch Jackson play rugby. It was a cold, drizzly Saturday afternoon and I was glad she was wearing the warm clothes my youngest sisters had taken her to buy. 'Mum loves the jacket (didn't we do well, Kate) and wore it out to lunch with us today, very cosy,' Ginny emailed after their joint shopping trip. 'She also wore my thermal tights that I thought she'd like to try on for size but she ended up wearing them all day. So after lunch we went to Postie Plus and bought her two pairs for herself, some warm socks and a hat. She is as snug as a bug.'

This email reminds me of the problem with memoir. Not only does it portray the world from a single point of view, but it also overstates the writer's role in that world. For every visit I made to Mum, each of my Wellington sisters made another. For every time I took her out, rubbed her back, calmed her fears, handled her crises and confusion, they did the same, or more, or something else.

Standing on the footpath outside Evans Bay Park, I gathered the hood of Mum's new jacket around her hollow cheeks. She hooked her fingers through the wire netting and peered through. I wondered what she made of the young men crashing about on the cut-up turf. She'd never shown the slightest interest in our national sport, or any sport for that matter. Gardening contained all the ingredients that fed her soul: creativity, beauty, exertion, solitude.

She didn't seem to notice when Jackson grounded the ball over the line but it was hard to distinguish one mud-streaked body from another. As soon as the game finished, I hurried her back to the car out of the biting wind and sent him a text: 'Gma and I were there. Nice try.'

'Tell him he has great legs,' she said.

That night I talked to Petra, whose house we were staying at while our renovations dragged on — a clear breach of Mum's three-day visitor rule. Petra knew the territory: I'd watched her run between two cities juggling sick parents, teenage boys and a full-time job. We agreed there had to be a better option than rattling around in our big houses or moving into a rest home as we aged. We imagined pooling our resources, buying a building and dividing it into small apartments with shared spaces and a nurse on hand. It sounds like a retirement village, I know, but we envisaged something small and intimate, with soul. Her partner, who'd designed our new kitchen, could draw up the plans.

It wouldn't be straightforward. We'd have to move out of our family home while we were still able in body and mind. We'd need a spare bedroom for the grandkids. Pat would insist on a garden and didn't want to live in the inner city. I'd want somewhere to write. Even so, I knew I'd be willing to make concessions so I didn't end up like Mum, alone in a house unsuited to her needs, unable to comprehend being happy anywhere else.

ROSE AND MIKE met with Carol, the Alzheimers Wellington manager, to discuss taking Mum to live with them. Then Rose arranged for the rest of us to meet her too. Over lunch at Kate's house, I felt like a surly teenager. I'd been grateful to Carol for confirming our suspicions that Mum had dementia but I didn't need to be hearing more bad news about her brain.

For someone who prides herself on asking questions, I'd done little research into the disease that was dominating our lives: I didn't know my amygdala from my hippocampus or my pre-frontal cortex. Today whole websites are devoted to the subject. There are online courses and blogs for carers and sufferers, endless information about how to avoid dementia and how to manage it. You can do a peanut butter smell test to see if you've got it, and take a virtual reality tour to experience life through the eyes of someone who has. (I'd never dare. What if it felt like my life now?)

A decade ago all that information wasn't around. Carol lent us a New Zealand memoir called *Dilemma of Dementia: A Daughter's Story*, Julia Millen's sad account of bringing her mother with Alzheimer's disease home to live with her in the 1980s. I found the personal letters and emails the most moving part, and was glad we were keeping ours.

To be fair, I didn't go looking for what else might be out there. There didn't seem much point. After Mum's CT scan showed cerebrovascular disease, there were no follow-up scans to track which parts of her brain were deteriorating and how her illness might progress. No definitive test to determine her level of dementia or rate of decline. No cure. The experts couldn't even agree whether drugs would help. Just getting through the here-and-now was hard enough without alarming myself about an uncertain future.

Anyway, academic articles about misfiring neurons and synapses, cells starved of oxygen and essential nutrients, reduced Mum to a damaged brain. Lists of symptoms never seemed to fit the mark. Mum could be difficult but she didn't swear or jumble her words, run away, put her shoes in the letterbox. The only way to be with Mum's dementia was to be with Mum: intelligent, irascible, hilarious, despondent, bewildered in her own unique way.

I don't remember discussing with Carol where Mum should live. What I do remember is her suggestion that we use something called 'therapeutic fibbing'. This meant telling Mum whatever was necessary to keep her calm, even if it wasn't factually correct. As soon as she got upset, her brain short-circuited and her behaviour got worse, Carol said. Mum wasn't capable of thinking things through logically; she didn't remember what we'd said — or indeed what she had either. What she retained was an emotional response.

So when she rang demanding her car keys, instead of telling her she didn't drive any more, we should offer to return them after dinner. When she said she needed to withdraw cash from the bank, instead of telling her we looked after her finances now, we should suggest going for a drive on the way. The important thing was to acknowledge the emotion behind Mum's demands (I've lost my independence, I'm worried about how I'm going to manage) rather than the demands themselves. Mum would soon forget about the car keys and the bank. She'd feel heard. We'd avoid a fight.

I was horrified. I'd spent my life trying to be upfront with people. Telling Mum the truth, however unpalatable, seemed essential to maintain her dignity. And then there was the dread of being found out. Mum's bullshit detector was finely tuned. If I lied to her, I was sure she'd know. Even if she forgot the details of my crime, a residual sense of having been deceived would linger.

On the other hand, I had to admit my truth-telling wasn't working. In spite of all my efforts to be straight with Mum, she was convinced I'd gone behind her back to the medical profession and the transport agency. Conflict clouded our time together. Responding honestly to her accusations only ramped up her rage. Both of us ended up seething and miserable.

My devotion to literal truth was also taking a hammering in

my creative writing workshop. My story about gang women was based on real-life events that had occurred three decades earlier. When I tried to evoke a scene, I couldn't recall the colour of the walls or the exact words of a conversation. What's more, the dozen women in the story each had their own perspective that didn't always gel with each other's or my own.

My classmates, a bevy of fiction writers, scoffed at my agonising about where, when, how and even if something actually happened. Hesitantly, I moved towards the concept of 'emotional truth' as my writing compass. This didn't mean I could make up events or pretend I'd felt one way when I'd felt another. But just as Carol was encouraging us to focus on the emotion behind Mum's demands, so too did I have to dig below the 'facts' of my story to reveal their essence.

For this, I needed imagination and flexibility: to recreate a scene around a single image or phrase that was seared into my brain, to concertina 30 years into 200 pages, to improvise details missing from my hazy visual sense and add inner thoughts I probably only framed later. Like a magpie, I scavenged for any trinket that would shine a light on the past. Even what I chose to leave out skewed the facts. Apparently Mark Twain called this 'lying towards the truth'. Literary therapeutic fibbing, if you will.

CHAPTER ELEVEN

ROLE MODELS

THE PAPER SELLOTAPED to the outside of Mum's front door read: 'PIP — please don't take my car without leaving a note and I don't want it left on the street when you return it — 2 neighbours have had trouble recently — and pop car keys through the (oops — there isn't one!) — you have a house key so leave on hall table.'

I screwed up the message, impressed with Mum's eloquence, amused at the non-existent letter flap, exasperated that her memory of the car remained lodged in her brain when everything else trickled out like water through a colander. In the dining room, one of the two new carers sat at the table polishing Mum's already-gleaming silver cutlery. Mum sat opposite, making no attempt to help. So far she seemed to be tolerating Jill, probably because they sneaked outside to smoke cigarettes together.

'Hi, I've brought your new pills,' I said. After talking to Carol, we'd decided to start Mum on the cognitive enhancer, Aricept. Anything that might give her remaining brain cells a boost was worth a try.

Mum's eyes narrowed. 'What new pills?'

'They're for your memory.' I lack the imagination for therapeutic fibbing. If I'd said they were for her wrinkles, Mum might have been delighted.

'What's wrong with my memory?'

I ignored the question and rummaged through the sideboard drawer looking for the cheque book she still commanded.

'Well, I'm not taking Fosamax any more,' Mum said. 'My GP says it causes cancer.' Fosamax was Mum's bone density drug, the one with the difficult instructions, the only one all the health professionals were adamant she should stay on.

'Well, your GP says these might help,' I said. 'They'd better cos they cost a bomb. I need you to reimburse me.' I put the cheque book in front of her and announced the hefty price tag, more than $200 a month.

'That's ridiculous,' Mum said.

Indeed. Aricept was unsubsidised in those days. I felt guilty about all the people who couldn't afford it, but it seemed like a double injustice to deprive Mum of a reprieve out of solidarity with the poor.

Mum's pen hovered above the blank cheque. Slowly she filled in the numbers I dictated and signed it. She ripped the cheque from the book but refused to hand it over.

Before I could stop Jill, she passed Mum the information leaflet from the Aricept packet, presumably to try and distract her.

Mum scanned the small print. 'Alzheimer's disease.' She spat out the words like a curse. 'The treating physician should evaluate the ability of patients to continue driving.'

My tongue got the better of me. 'Good thing you don't have to worry about that.'

'Yes, I do,' she said.

'No, Mum, you've lost your licence.'

'I'm allowed to drive to the supermarket.'

I shook my head from side to side, not trusting myself to speak.

Mum scowled and bent over the leaflet again. A smile twitched at the corners of her mouth. 'Do not use if pregnant until you have discussed with your pharmacist or doctor,' she read. She looked up. For a moment, the old twinkle was back in her eye.

ROSE PHONED IN tears. Mum had rung to say she'd had a bad dream about Dad. They'd been in Melbourne and he'd disappeared. Mum's voice was slurred, Rose said. She told Rose she'd been walking round the house but still couldn't find him. It wasn't clear if this was in the dream or after she woke up. We wondered if she'd had another mini-stroke.

In spite of our efforts, Mum was spending too much time alone. Someone told us about The Chelsea Club, which provided respite care for people with Alzheimer's disease and dementia. Within minutes of meeting the manager, Barb, who knew of our family through Catholic circles, I wanted to hug her. Everything she said about their service felt extraordinary in its ordinariness.

The club operated out of a homely old villa in Lyall Bay. Four paid staff and volunteers, all trained, looked after up to 12 clients a day who were known as members. The terms 'dementia' and 'memory loss' were never used. Members got a cooked midday meal, morning and afternoon tea, activities and an outing. Best of all, they were picked up and dropped off. We wouldn't have to deal with Mum's protests at either end of the day.

When Capital Coast Health approved one day of respite care a week for Mum, Barb rang her and invited her to join the club. Mum thanked her and declined. She wasn't lonely, she said; she had lots of friends and family popping in. A little nonplussed,

Barb went round to Colville Street, where she helped Mum sweep some leaves before suggesting they go for a drive. Mum locked the house and hopped into Barb's car. We were too relieved to ponder whether this meant she'd go off with anyone who showed an interest in her garden.

Rose had dinner with Mum after her first club day. 'We chatted about the balloon games etc and how wonderful everyone else was (including the other non-staff)', Rose emailed. For Mum to think she was a staff member was less improbable than her playing balloon games. She'd spent her whole life doing good works in the community and, although she shared the pallor and cloudy eyes of the other members, she looked in better nick than most.

'She thinks they do a wonderful job and "it's all charity",' Rose continued. 'But she is cross that the GP told this Barbara that she was lonely and that's why she was 'invited' and she really doesn't want to join the club and certainly doesn't want to go every week. Once a month — maybe.'

The following week, Mum turned the Chelsea Club volunteer away in the morning but relented when the van came back to take her on the afternoon drive. The week after that, she sent Barb a letter saying she was no longer able to attend because of family commitments.

It was the first written resignation the club had ever received, Barb told me. 'Rosaleen's a strong woman, isn't she?'

I felt a flash of surprise, followed by pride. Dad had always been the strong one — at least till he got sick and Mum had to make decisions for both of them. Even then, her power often came from her passivity. She got her way not by confrontation but by clamming up or digging in her heels. Many's the time I'd become outraged on her behalf, only to have her undermine my efforts. Now she was getting outraged all by herself.

For all its frustration and sorrow, dementia brought out a directness in Mum, an underlying strength of will. Like a toddler whose wild unreasonableness is a thrilling expression of spirit, except when it's directed at you, there was something admirable about this new mother who'd finally learned to say no.

MUM DIDN'T HAVE far to look for feisty female role models. On her father's side, her great-grandmother Catherine Brown was orphaned in England, married her first husband Herri Waigth in Australia, lost him and two babies, and moved to New Zealand in 1864.

She had two more husbands, owned property in and out of Roxburgh, and became one of the oldest hotel keepers in the district at a time when women were not allowed to be licensees. When she died, her will was published in the local paper. It left her third husband a glass of beer a day for the rest of his life 'cos that's about all he was worth', Des told me the day I recorded his and Mum's memories.

Mum's maternal grandmother, Mary McErlane, emigrated from County Derry, Ireland, in 1877 at the age of 22. Four years later, according to her obituary in the *New Zealand Tablet*, she married John Kearney, who'd 'taken up' a piece of swampy land where 'after hard toil, industry and perseverance, they carved a home for themselves out of the wilderness of scrub, maori heads [the name settlers gave to snow tussock] and tussock which is today one of the most beautiful homes on the Maniototo Plain'.

This was Springfield, the Ranfurly farm on which Mum's mother Dolly and her three sisters grew up. When their brother John went off to war, the girls milked the cows and helped with the stock, Des said. This didn't sound at all like Mum, who was scared of mice, and one year left the Christmas goose hanging in the Roxburgh coal shed till it 'putrefied' because she couldn't bear to pluck and dress it after Dolly had to go into hospital.

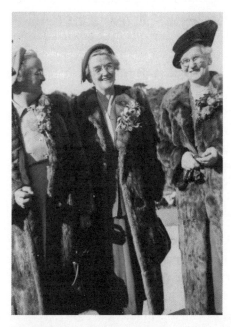

left
The Kearney girls in their furs and finery. My grandmother Mary Rose, known as Dolly, flanked by her sisters Vera (left) and Sarah. The close-knit trio ventured as far afield together as the Melbourne Cup and Fiji.

———

below
3 Melrose Street, the Roxburgh house where Mum grew up.

———

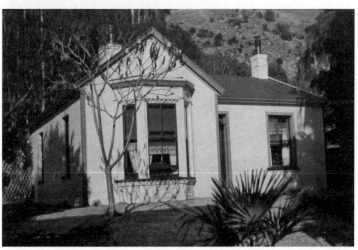

Mary, the obituary went on to say, 'had a very genial and kindly disposition and wherever she went was the life and soul of the party — young and old'. She died in 1921 — of a broken heart, it was said — after John survived the war only to be taken in the flu epidemic on the way home.

In Mum's childhood, Mary's oldest daughter Sarah was 'the boss, she ran the show'; she even named Mum and Des when they were born. Sarah and her husband owned the draper's shop in Roxburgh. On Saturday nights they'd go to the pictures where all the children sat up the front. 'And if there was any sort of disturbance from the front row, she would just lean over with her umbrella, or her walking stick it might have been, and bonk them on the head,' Mum said.

This story sparked another. Sarah always wore a fox fur, complete with the head. 'And I do remember, you make me remember, we would be at Mass and maybe I was fidgeting a bit, and there was a little thing that you did and the teeth would snap at you, and all she had to do was that and I was' — Mum sat up straight and folded her arms — 'perfect behaviour.'

The second Kearney girl, Kate, was generally missing from the family folklore, perhaps because 'the marriage was pretty slippery', and she moved away from her sisters. As a teenager, Mum was shocked by the poverty her aunt was living in when Sarah took her to visit Kate in Gisborne. 'All I can remember is a lean-to at the back and some coal-fired cooking arrangement and her cooking us a meal on it.' Sarah intervened and took Kate back to Roxburgh for some time.

Third in line was Dolly, our grandmother, as gentle as her younger sister Vera was gruff. Vera petrified us — and Mum — as children. But the more I heard about my great-aunt, the more I liked the sound of the staunch Labour supporter who lived in Waimate and stood up to her conservative Roxburgh rellies. One of the first women to drive a car, she once wrestled a stray lamb into the boot and took it home, Des said. She and Dad sparred constantly. One Christmas she sent him a single sock; the next Christmas he sent it back. The year after that, it was a turnip.

All the Kearney girls 'could tell the most outrageous lies with the straightest face', Mum said. This applied even to my adored grandmother, I discovered when I got the hiccups on a family drive as a child. They wouldn't stop. Suddenly Grandma addressed me in the sternest voice I'd ever heard her use: 'Phillipa, did you take my silver teapot?'

I froze mid-*hic*, first in shock that she'd think I might steal from her, then in shame when the carload erupted in laughter that her trick had worked. After Mum died, Des sent me the silver teapot from Australia. It should stay in the family, he said. I tried to palm it off on my sisters but no one wanted it. I still eye it on the shelf with suspicion.

'DO WE HAVE any time frame for moving Mum? I don't want to appear pushy, but she is really losing it at the moment,' Ginny emailed after she found Mum writing lists of days she claimed the carers hadn't shown up, most of them in the future. Reluctantly we began to visit retirement villages and rest homes, although it still seemed out of the question that she'd ever live in any of them.

In the carpark of one, I ran into an acquaintance, a journalist. For a minute I wondered if he was doing an exposé of aged care. Then he told me his mother had died in the dementia unit and he was there to get her things. 'Don't put your mother in here,' he said. 'It's awful.'

He offered to meet up. It was the first time I'd talked to someone who'd been through a similar ordeal to us. Like Mum, his mother had vascular dementia. She too had lived alone in the family home for a long time, supported by her children who made a pact not to move her without her permission, even after she started having hallucinations. One day, in a brief, lucid moment, she agreed to go into care: something I couldn't imagine Mum ever doing.

'How long was your mother sick?' I asked, meaning, *How long will this go on for? How bad will it get?*

'Five years,' he said. 'That's how long it usually is with vascular dementia.' I was surprised by his certainty but I knew he'd have done his homework. I cast my mind back, trying to pinpoint the onset of the disease for Mum. Was it two years earlier, when she and Des travelled south to visit their relations? Or the following year when she made multiple batches of tamarillo chutney, cleaned her teeth in front of Pat, duplicated my salad, transformed her calendar into a kaleidoscope? Or was it later again, as the geriatrician insisted — when she failed the driving test — in which case we were only just out of the starting blocks?

The fact is, disaster doesn't always announce itself with a drumroll. Sometimes it sneaks up, like time itself, lulling us into a false sense that nothing has changed. If Dad had been alive, he'd have picked up the signs sooner. If Mum had been less capable, she couldn't have hidden them for so long. For us, her children, dementia began as a scrambled message here, a missed appointment there, some confusion, irritability, withdrawal, dwelling in the past. *Just part of getting older*, you tell yourself. Until one day, your growing unease that all is not well becomes the crushing knowledge that the mother you thought you knew has gone and she is never coming back.

CHAPTER TWELVE

———

WISE OLD WOMAN

From: Matt
To: Rose; Ginny; Pip; Kate; Liz
Sent: Monday, July 10, 2006 09:34 AM
Subject: A day in the life

Hi y'all,
Spent a lovely afternoon with Mum yesterday. Yes she was
complaining of diarrhoea, and yes she (thought she) had
cancelled her hairdresser appointment. So we just flopped
on the couches, and ate (lots of) chicken soup and French
bread, and never went to the toilet once — either of us.

We talked about how Pip got to Roxburgh when she was a
toddler, and how she could know that Grandma had fed her
with a salt spoon. We talked about the blackout curtains
at her college, and how people in the south never really

believed the Japanese were coming. We rang the woman in Dunedin who wrote months ago to interview Mum for her history of Pregnancy Help. She told me how difficult it has been since Ginny walked off with her phone list (you have to nail things down when that Ginny's in the house!!). Then, when we found the phone list next to the phone, she told me how Ginny must have snuck it back in.

We put the new cheque book in the top right-hand drawer of the desk, cut up the old bankcard, and put the new book of taxi chits in her handbag . . . which had been missing all morning, but someone (Ginny?) must have returned beside her chair. We talked about Liz being in England, and why Rose was late for lunch, and even about Matt coming home in November. We fixed the broken TV and CD player.

I was thinking that she is in a process of getting us all sorted. No matter how outrageous her various accusations are, there's probably some fundamental truth/memory underlying them. (And there's so little anger in them this time.) I was thinking how I'm always the one who gets a mention when the question of borrowing money off her comes up. We could probably develop a family archetypology based on a wise old woman's half-memories:

Matt — the one who's always broke and borrowing money.

Ginny — the one who's always using other people's things (and the one who's so good at fixing things — so practical).

Pip — the one who's always stopping her doing things (and the essential one — maybe the external controller we all need when we can't quite trust ourselves?).

Rose — the reliable one (though where was she for lunch?). I haven't quite got you taped yet, but it's something about being a fixed point in an unpredictable world.

Liz — the unflappable one (does this mean Liz that we're in a rehearsal for when you are 70?).

Kate — the one who just does her own thing. No rhyme or reason, and no expectation that rhymes or reasons should be applied.

Yesterday, at least, I found Mum much calmer than when I was home in Feb. We didn't get onto the photo-albums but I think that's what she'd really like to talk about.

It will be lovely to catch up with some of you tonight for Ginny's birthday.

Matt

Not everyone would describe a person with dementia as a wise old woman operating from a fundamental truth. But I agreed with the box Matt thought Mum had put me in, though not the lack of anger attached to it. It was as if she'd turned me into Dad, an authority figure who decided what was best for her. I'm not convinced she formed this opinion after she got dementia; I suspect she just felt freer to express it. That's why I couldn't accept people's advice not to take her personal attacks to heart, that it wasn't my mother talking, that it was the disease. It was always my mother talking. Only now her shadow side — the darkness that hides within us all — was on the rise.

Mum and I had a rocky start. All the signs are that she was exhausted by repeated pregnancies, isolated, not naturally maternal. Her depletion led to mine. In my childhood memories, she's a shadowy figure, distant and put-upon, her touch practical rather than tender. No matter how long I keep my eyes closed, I can't feel her arms around me, sense her hand brush my cheek or her lips on my forehead. She was always busy, morning to night. Of course she was. So many of us, so little back-up. But it was more than that, I think. If she sat down, she might never get up. If she stopped to think, she might doubt the point of it all. If she let us in, she might sink under the weight of so many small bodies.

Don't get me wrong. Childhood photos reveal a bright-eyed, well-fed bunch. After my early eating difficulties, I thrived in the middle of my family: a tomboy fond of walking on my hands and shimmying up the inside of the door frame where I'd perch, legs braced on either side, until Mum told me to *get down from there*. When I contemplate Ginny's orphaned beginnings and the harrowing childhoods of many of the gang women I know, it seems ludicrous to find fault with my own. There was food and money, safety and laughter, friends and holidays. Dad provided the rules and the warmth, Mum the steadfastness that kept us afloat.

But wait. Matt says it was Mum who provided his warmth; Kate says Mum chose to be a wife and mother. Which makes me think about other possibilities. Could there be more to Mum's early married life than the exhaustion of motherhood and the sadness of moving an island away from her own mother? Perhaps the girl who'd outshone the boys in debating was excited to be heading to the capital with her clever husband. (By 30, Dad had been a lecturer in pathology at the University of Otago for three years and had just been offered a partnership with a respected Wellington pathologist.)

Certainly Mum had no time for small-town nosiness. When Dad wrote away for Tex Morton's guitar manual at the Roxburgh Hydro camp, she insisted it come in plain brown wrapping. What the new GP did in his spare time was no one else's business.

In Wellington, Mum somehow found the inner strength and outer resources to recover from her quick-fire foursome. The church that had got her into this pickle now came to her aid. Dad's aunt, Sister Kevin, took Matt into her infant class at St Mary's College before he was four. On his first school report, she gave him 100 per cent in all subjects, along with the comment, 'A genius — like his father.'

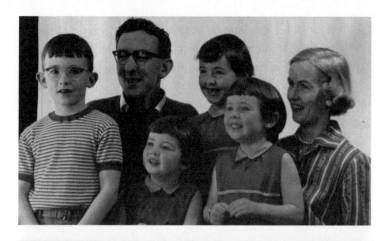

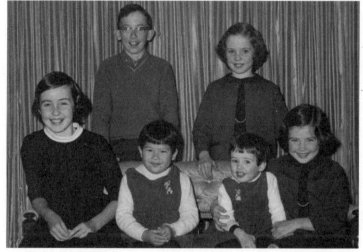

above
Mum and Dad and their quick-fire foursome, around 1959. Liz, Rose and
I are wearing matching 'zebra dresses', sewn by Mum, with a black-
and-white-striped skirt and trim. Matt's t-shirt completes the theme.

———

below
Ginny joined our family as a toddler in 1963, followed by
Kate three months later. Standing: Matt and me. Sitting, from
left: Liz, Ginny, Kate, Rose. Note the matching outfits.

———

Two years later, she took Liz at four and two-thirds. Mum had a brief respite after she packed Rose off to school before she found herself with a toddler and a new baby, starting all over again.

Catholic connections also brought us Mary McCabe to help Mum with the housework. She was tiny, with a wizened face and a broad Irish brogue. Not much cleaning got done, I fear, but Mary filled our mouths with lollies and our heads with tales of the little people. When she did get out the ironing board, she set it up low enough for a leprechaun, to make us laugh. We loved her; it seemed possible she'd sprung from under a toadstool herself.

GROWING UP, I had little interest in the household drudgery that filled my mother's days. It was my dashing, driven father I adored, with his healing hands and nose like Henry Kissinger's. When he was around (never enough), he played games, took us on picnics (provided by Mum), imbued in us his love of the sea. At night, he read us stories about Eloise, Madeleine and Pippi Longstocking — fearless, irrepressible girls without a mother between them — and sang us to sleep on his guitar with 'The Fox Went Out on a Winter's Night' and 'Oh My Darling Clementine'. In our college years, he helped us write speeches for drama and debating (Mum never let on about her own talent in this area) and encouraged us to express our opinions — until they conflicted with his.

Dad provided the hugs. The discipline too: I rarely remember being smacked but he commanded absolute obedience. Even the advice on women's matters came from my understanding medical father. It was him I confided in when I got my period, Mum who some months later handed me a box of tampons and told me to read the instructions. Liz found me weeping in the bathroom and showed me what to do with them.

But that doesn't do Mum justice either. While Dad talked

passionately about family, I came to realise it was Mum who knew how to 'do' family. When she first came to Wellington, she told me, she couldn't believe that no one invited Dad's maiden aunts home after Mass on Sundays. On her watch, relations were rounded up, along with the priest and assorted others. As a teenager I often despaired at the hotchpotch of people I had to entertain in the lounge while Mum cooked up a storm in the kitchen.

When I delve into my memory, other images surface of her love in action: Mum as the sole audience at one of our interminable puppet shows, providing lemonade at half-time. Mum bearing a tray of ginger gems and cocoa into the lounge so we could have Sunday tea by the fire in our jarmies. Mum taking Liz, Rose and me as little girls to Roxburgh, a marathon by ferry and road that required an overnight stay in a guest house.

When we arrived, Grandma's house reeked of lamb's tongue being boiled for dinner. After I'd gagged on the slimy pink slices for a while, one of them (if I have to pick, it's Mum, surprisingly) let me off and I scuttled from the table in disgrace.

On that trip we all wore tartan skirts with white bodices. If we'd been younger, we'd have been decked out in the matching dresses she sewed us: tulip dresses, zebra dresses, sailor dresses, bib frocks. I'm sure I got the lead role as Snow White at primary school because of the elaborate costumes she could run up. I was hopeless at sewing, myself. At college, I'd sneak home my half-finished shorty pyjamas and A-line skirt for her to fix the elastic and put the zip in. She'd get out her Bernina, never questioning the ethics of doing it for me, nor enquiring how I was going to sneak them back into my cubbyhole without being caught and rapped across the knuckles with the sewing scissors by Sister Regina.

Mum never taught me to sew — perhaps I didn't show enough interest. But during my short-lived Girl Guide career, I was annoyed when she made me practise the correct way to tuck in sheet corners before she'd vouch for my bed-making skills. The reason became clear the day I recorded her memories. On her first night as a scared, homesick boarder at St Dom's, she had to make her own bed, she told me. 'Sister Winefride was having a conniption on the sideline and she said, "Don't you know how to make a bed?" and I said "No". So she gave me a lesson on how to make a bed that I have never forgotten.' Mum wasn't going to let any daughter of hers be shown up like that.

I asked Mum if she'd been close to her mother, Dolly. 'Well, you see, I wasn't there, so teenage years were just any old years,' she said, side-stepping the question. And later: 'We went to boarding school. Never went home again.' This wasn't strictly true — Mum returned to Roxburgh for school holidays and to support her mother after her father died — but the early wrench must have felt definitive. I wondered how it had affected Mum's own mothering. Or more likely, I didn't wonder then, it just occurs to me now.

ELEGANT AS MUM was, she didn't pass on her sense of style to her daughters. Unless you count the dress-up box. It wasn't a box, it was a tin trunk, full of her gorgeous cast-offs that we were allowed to wear on special occasions. In a letter to an aunt when I was 11, I wrote that I was going to a party in 'that Chinese dressing gown which Daddy brought Mummy from Australia . . . that looks like an evening dress', and 'the high heels which Mummy wore when she was a hostess in the ball; those glittering silver ones'.

Even then, I'd have cringed at my babyish use of 'Mummy' and refused to call her that in front of my friends. But she hated us calling her 'Mum'. It was coarse, she said. So was eating in the street, chewing gum anywhere, putting your elbows on the table and burping. She was big on manners.

When it came to fashion, Mum's main guidance was on how

to keep things in. At college, she gave me a girdle to flatten my stomach; in the days before pantyhose, it had suspenders to attach my stockings to. Later, in my first flush of feminism, she took me aside and told me some women could get away without wearing a bra, but I wasn't one of them.

For all the female energy in our house, we were never girly girls. In spite of all the tubes and potions on her dressing table, Mum never showed us the womanly arts. This was not entirely her fault. Keeping his five daughters out of moral danger weighed heavily on Dad.

Ginny and Kate may have had an easier time of it, as the youngest often do, but Liz, Rose and I went through as a job lot under his regime. Mascara, jeans and bikinis were forbidden (too provocative). We didn't own a TV. When Dad occasionally hired one for the holidays, he banned us from watching the classic 1960s pop show *C'mon* because of its raunchy, half-clad, go-go dancers. Comics were also forbidden (lazy reading, subversive), as were Weetbix and Marmite (Sanitarium, i.e. Seventh Day Adventist infidels).

At the same time, like many kids of our generation, we had a great deal of freedom. By the time I was eight or nine, we roamed the Tinakori Hills from our home in Thorndon without adult supervision. And during those Waikanae family holidays, we'd disappear for hours on the bikes Dad hired for us, returning only for meals. The moment we turned 15, he taught each of us to drive, a strategy that paid off when there was a string of chauffeurs to ferry him when he couldn't drive himself.

At his best, Dad was a man for all seasons, equally comfortable serving the homeless at the soup kitchen, talking to my gang friends, or leading a conference of Catholic doctors. An independent thinker, he leaned towards National but voted Social Credit several times, and Labour when Norm Kirk promised state aid to Catholic schools.

He loved gadgets. We may have been the last family in the

neighbourhood to get TV but we were the first to get a dishwasher. Numerous other mod cons were purchased 'for Mum' to make her life easier: a clothes dryer, an ironing machine, a leaf sweeper, a Busy Bee floor polisher for the gold-and-white lino hallway at Wadestown Road that was the length of a cricket pitch and showed every mark and scuff. Dad also had an impossibly steep driveway extension built up to the house so Mum could unload the groceries at the front door.

Some of his solicitude may have stemmed from guilt. As I got older, I picked up on Mum's resentment at Dad's absence. He was on 35 medical and church committees, chair of 18 at one point, she claimed, including running marriage guidance courses throughout the parish while she spent another evening alone at home.

All this changed when Dad got sick. I was 16, beginning to think for myself. In his illness, he clung to his Maker just as I started to question both of them. 'Don't upset your father or —' became Mum's mantra. She didn't need to finish the sentence: the burden of being responsible for another dreadful seizure froze me in my teenage angst. It also left me in no-man's land. To reject Dad's God meant losing my father. To accept his God meant losing myself. And there I stayed.

Dad's brain tumour brought me closer to Mum. Although she threw out almost everything personal, she kept two letters I wrote to her: one in 1976 after I left university, the other in 1981, the year I became a mother. In both I say how much I value her love and friendship. In the first, I exhort her to tell me 'exactly what the situation is with Dad, even if it does look rather gloomy'. In the second, with rather more self-awareness, I apologise for cutting her off whenever she starts to share her feelings. 'I get frightened when you are upset,' I say. 'Part of it is not wanting to face Dad's illness and part is not wanting to face your sorrow.' This reminds me that Mum suppressed her emotions not only to protect herself but also to spare her children.

When I had my own kids, the pair of us would regularly head off to an evening movie, followed by a glass of wine and a sly cigarette. I like to think the confiding went both ways on these occasions, although no doubt I hogged the conversation. Mum was a superb listener and, if I'm honest, I probably thought my life was more interesting than hers — and she let me.

Not any more. As the ground crumbled beneath her, her needs became more visible, her demands vocal — as if she'd outlined them in bold with the same felt-tip markers she used to highlight the entries on her calendar.

CHAPTER THIRTEEN

—

LADYLIKE
BEHAVIOUR

THANKS TO ROSE, who'd taken it upon herself to chivvy Mum out of the bath and into the volunteer's car every Wednesday morning, we still had a foot in the door of the Chelsea Club. There was something about their warm, down-to-earth service that stopped Mum saying a definitive no, as she did to almost everything else.

'Her voice was strong and "buzzy" — not weary at all,' Rose emailed after phoning Mum one evening. 'When prompted, she told me she'd been at Chelsea Club. When prompted again, agreed she'd gone out to Southward Car Museum. She said — and I write it here as evidence: "I never regret going. I always enjoy it." Yay — go the Chelsea Buns.' So when Capital Coast Health agreed to fund a second day of respite care a week, we accepted. Anything had to be better than Mum's mad activity at Colville

Street, obsessing about her affairs and shouting at the carers.

It was good to know she was getting fed at the Chelsea Club, too. She didn't eat properly on her own, even when we left her meals. It was hard to know if she forgot, had lost her appetite, felt sick, or needed company.

I went round to cook her dinner at Colville Street. Afterwards we went through to the lounge with our cups of tea. Mum sat on the couch, her matchstick legs crossed in that ladylike way of hers: knees slanted to the side, right leg snaking around the left. 'Don't, you'll get varicose veins!' she'd warn when I tried to mimic her as a child. She'd had to go into hospital to have hers stripped and spent a whole summer wearing thick compression stockings.

Tonight she was smiley and chatty and funny, and I realised how much I'd been dreading the visit — and what good company she used to be. I wondered if the new dementia drug was helping her mood, if not her confusion. I got up to do the dishes and asked if she'd finished her tea. She handed it to me with an inch of dregs. 'A lady never drains her cup,' she said.

Mum had spent her whole life learning to be a lady. There's a photo of her, five or six years old, clambering up a narrow dirt track to the Roxburgh power house, one of her father's schemes to bring electricity to the region. She's out with her mother Dolly, her Aunt Vera and a neighbour. The women are all in their Sunday best including good shoes, scarves and furs. Mum has a miniature fur flung around her neck too. Her Aunt Sarah would have given it to her, she said. 'She did dress me up a bit, not having any little girls of her own.'

I asked Mum what else a lady didn't do. 'A lady never eats more than three pieces,' she recited in a sing-song voice. Dolly had passed on this rule of etiquette as they walked home after a sumptuous afternoon tea at Mrs Dunlay's, her mother's friend. Mum was a teenager, back from St Dom's for the holidays.

'Had you pigged out?' I asked, inconceivable as it seemed that her hollow cheeks had ever been filled with food.

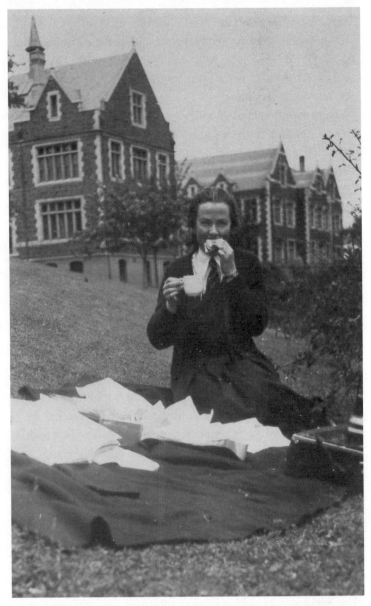

'A lady never drains her cup': Mum in the grounds of St Dominic's College, Dunedin, where she was a boarder for five years in the 1940s.

Mum stared into the fire.

I repeated the question.

'Probably,' she said vaguely. Her grip seemed to be slipping not just on the present but also on the past. She'd set off down memory lane only to pull up around the first corner as if mist had rolled across the road and obscured her view. Previously she'd have told me that Dolly's advice came after Mum admitted she'd eaten 13 pieces at that afternoon tea. As a child, I too had been taken to Mrs Dunlay's and endured an afternoon of women's gossip in return for a vast array of club sandwiches, asparagus rolls, cheese puffs, pikelets with cream and jam, cinnamon oysters, melting moments, neenish tarts, cakes on tiered stands — enough to feed the town. For Mum, used to a diet of wartime boarding school stodge, it must have been irresistible.

Somehow she emerged from college a plump 13 stone. At meals, she told me the day I recorded her memories — when she was still so eloquent — she sat next to Patricia Sim who was 'the leanest thing I've ever seen, the tallest, skinniest. I used to give her those terrible steamed puddings and blancmange. I couldn't stand all this bread with something scraped on it, it wouldn't have been butter. So she used to eat my share. And as I got fatter, she got thinner. I didn't eat anything. I put on so much weight. It must have been just sheer routine, I think.'

The weight fell off Mum as soon as she left college, and it stayed off. None of her adult daughters' waists were ever tiny enough to fit the pale green-and-lemon chiffon ball gown that transformed our mother of six into a princess as she disappeared into the night on Dad's arm in a cloud of perfumed loveliness.

A LADY CURBED her appetite. A lady curbed her emotions, too. That night at Mum's, I lingered, savouring the warmth of the fire and her mood. As we chatted, I mentioned that a friend's daughter was going through a hard time. Mum remarked that her own life had been easy.

'I don't think there's anything easy about looking after a sick husband for twenty-five years,' I said.

It was as if I'd hit a geyser. Mum uncrossed her legs and leaned her elbows on her thighs. Her frail body began to tremble violently. 'It was awful,' she whispered. 'And the noise.' She meant when Dad had a *grand mal*. She watched him constantly, she said. Trying to anticipate the next fit. Listening for sounds in the night. Never letting down her guard. Year after year, until he died.

A picture of a family meal flashed through my mind: Dad at one end of the oval dining table, Mum at the other, her fork poised halfway to her mouth as he crashed from his chair. Her look of horror as he lay at our feet, first rigid, then jerking and shaking and growling from a place no one could reach him. Time stopped. No one spoke.

At last, he came back to us, dazed and spent. If she'd known how, Mum might have got down on her knees and cradled his head in her lap. But she was too appalled and frightened — and so were we.

Seeing her rock back and forth on the humpty, I realised Mum's body had absorbed the physical trauma of Dad's seizures she'd witnessed. But it was only when I read Scottish journalist Sally Magnusson's *Where Memories Go*, about caring for her mother with Alzheimer's disease, that I considered their possible effect on Mum's brain. Looking for causes of her mother's illness, Magnusson came across an Edinburgh University study that linked dementia with 'elevated psychological distress', even decades later, particularly if it was suppressed. Her mother had lost a son when he was 12 and been unable to grieve his death, she said.

In *When the Body Says No*, Canadian physician and author Gabor Maté explores this idea further. He says emotional repression creates stress that can make our bodies break down, often in the form of autoimmune diseases like multiple sclerosis and rheumatoid arthritis (Mum was suspected of having the latter after Dad died). There's growing evidence that Alzheimer's disease also comes into this category, he says.

The immediate cause of Mum's vascular dementia was high blood pressure that led to mini-strokes that starved her brain of oxygen. But, like Sally Magnusson's mother, Mum supressed her distress about Dad's brain tumour for decades, as her shaking body showed. This was partly due to her upbringing. She never heard her parents raise their voices or disagree, she told me. 'In front of us, anyway. It was always harmonious and happy.' Making a fuss was not in her repertoire.

Our western view of illness must also take some responsibility. How different Mum's reaction might have been if society had seen Dad's seizures as an honour, not a scourge. Some cultures do. As Ann Fadiman describes in her remarkable book *When the Spirit Catches You, You Fall Down,* the Hmong people of Laos believe epilepsy is a sign that someone is spiritually gifted. Imagine if Dad had gained the status of tohunga, holy man, rather than invalid, after he got sick. Imagine if Mum had been revered as his caregiver instead of feeling terrified and ashamed. After Dad's massive first seizure — the one that nearly killed him — her blood pressure skyrocketed. Not properly treated, this led to her dementia. Unfair as it seems, her illness was born out of his.

By the time Dad died, Mum's emotions were frozen. I did enough crying for both of us. It annoyed her. In the weeks after his death, she wouldn't let me stand next to her when we gathered: she couldn't stand the silent waterfall running down my face. I wished I could stop for both our sakes — but I was desolate. My anchor was gone. Even worse, the tug-of-war between my father's love for me and for his God would never be resolved. I wonder if Mum felt the same about his love for her.

'You think too much,' I hear her say.

WE DISCOVERED THAT Mum was eligible for half-price taxi fares and hastily signed her up. The whiff of freedom sparked what remained of the 86 billion neurons in her brain and she got the hang of them immediately. Rose gave her the phone number of a friend, a cab driver, to call if she wanted to go anywhere. Mum got on better with him than with her carers.

Perhaps he could take over, Liz suggested, tongue-in-cheek. 'He can sit outside in the car so Mum doesn't have to talk to him or make him cups of tea when she doesn't feel like it but be available for trips. We'd have to pay him a retainer — what's it cost for 2 mornings care/week + taxis. What d'ya reckon? I wonder if he could do her pills? :)'

Liz's flight of fancy didn't seem much madder than anything else we'd tried. After Mum complained the latest carer was unreliable and 'a law unto herself', Ginny and I arranged to meet the woman. We discovered she was the primary breadwinner in her family and had seven other clients, some with more advanced dementia than Mum's; that her husband was about to donate a kidney to their daughter who was on dialysis; and that the daughter and her 10-year-old son lived with them as well. It was a miracle she turned up to look after Mum at all.

Mum's six hours' homecare a week, including admin costs, took out half her pension: the agency was too new for clients to qualify for government subsidies. It paid its carers above average, which we applauded. Still, it was barely a living wage for the women — and they were all women — who traipsed from house to house, providing the invisible support that kept old people in the community. Back then, they weren't trained in dementia care. Some had more empathy than others, but Mum rebuffed them all.

I don't know if someone exceptional could have got through her defences. Looking at the agency's website today, I feel a pang of envy at the photos of smiling clients leaning against carers next to appreciative testimonials: 'I have three charming and interesting women sharing the hours to prepare an evening meal 3 times a week. This meal is always delicious.'

I can't imagine Mum ever saying that, especially about food cooked by a stranger. Her nausea had become persistent. 'Left Mum today lying on the couch with a wheat bag to her tummy listening to Nat King Cole — it was a hard thing to do,' Kate emailed. Then, with her nurse's eye, she added, 'I'm actually quite concerned about the state of her bowels, or more importantly the state of her nutritional absorption. Couldn't find any Immodium (which I hate her taking anyway) but Ginny's going to pop in and follow up tomorrow. And please push the water, everyone.'

Mum still enjoyed talking about food. Come springtime, when Pat and I were finally back in our house, she sat at the picnic table and watched him mound soil around his seed potatoes. The two of them drooled at the prospect of new spuds smothered with butter and mint for Christmas dinner.

I went inside and Mum followed me. While I made lunch, she read out recipes from an Annabel Langbein cookbook, and ticked a few. 'For you to make later,' she said.

Once upon a time, the ticks would have been for her. Good food ran in her blood. Even on family picnics, Dolly would serve roast chicken and vegetables, kept warm in a thermo-jug, on china plates with serviettes, followed by trifle, fruit salad and whipped cream.

Every day at primary school in Roxburgh, Mum and Des went home to a hot midday meal and dessert. 'We were like the ducks, all we had to do was walk across the road.'

Secretly Mum envied the railway workers' children who came on the school bus and gobbled their sandwiches in the playground, including her 'very best friend' Jacqueline Parker. 'The Parkers weren't actually railway children but they lived in the railway settlement,' she said. 'And there were twelve of them.

I used to think it was terrific to go to their house, it was just so full of people and activity.'

AFTER MUM WENT to boarding school she never saw Jacqueline again. 'She probably left school and went to work in the jam factory,' she said. It was a world away from the University of Otago where Mum began a degree in home science after college. She moved into Dominican Hall, a girls' hostel run by the same sisters who'd run St Dom's, and later went flatting.

I'd always pictured home science as a sort of finishing school for future housewives where the lucky ones snared an aspiring doctor from the medical school, until historian Ali Clarke put me right. 'Home science did, to some extent, segregate capable women from the "pure" science courses, but it also offered them opportunities,' Clarke says in her excellent online history of the university. 'Degree students took advanced courses in chemistry, and many went on to become school teachers in the pure sciences as well as home economics.'

Mum was one of these students. After her father's sudden death in 1950, she cut short her final year's study to go back to Roxburgh and support her mother. For a while she taught home economics, possibly the only job she ever had outside the home apart from serving in her Aunt Sarah's draper's shop on Friday nights. She didn't enjoy teaching, although she didn't have long to find out. A year later she and Dad were married, and her family became the focus of her home science skills.

We four older kids had to eat everything on our plates with the exception of three personal 'dislikes'. (This rule had disappeared by the time Kate arrived; her early diet is said to have consisted of Chocolate Quik and bread and honey.) I can't remember my first dislike — swede or cucumber or perhaps the ghastly boiled

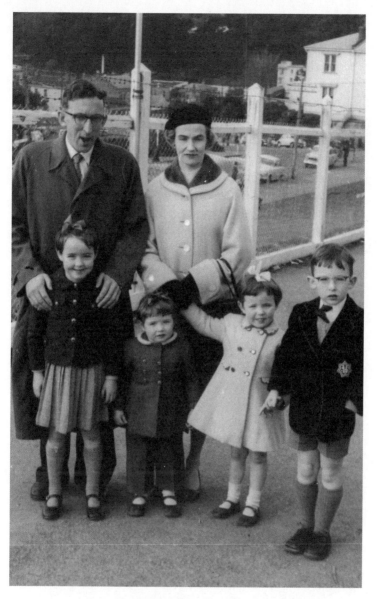

Mum and Dad with, from left, Liz, Rose, me and Matt outside the
Wellington Trade Fair, John Street, in the late 1950s. The fair became
an annual family outing although it was usually Dad who took us.

sheep's tongue — but Rose's was that childhood bane, Brussels sprouts. My second was a sickly jaffa pudding that I nominated after one mouthful and that Mum never made again. I was too scared to choose the third in case something worse came along.

Fortunately, Mum was a fabulous cook who served up spaghetti bolognese, pork chow mein, veal stroganoff and coleslaw long before they were mainstream. By the time I was a teenager, Graham Kerr, Hudson and Halls and Julia Childs sat alongside the *Edmonds Cookery Book* and *Triple Tested Recipe Book*. Mum's desserts were legendary: lemon meringue pie, chocolate log, those perfect pavlovas. Her tins were full of ginger biscuits, afghans, cinnamon-flavoured Belgian square with a layer of raspberry jam. And yet, I must confess, for years I swapped the meat sandwiches in my school lunch box for my friends' jam ones, and Mum's home baking for biscuits out of a packet.

In summertime, there was bottling: row upon row of tall glass jars filled with pears, Golden Queen peaches, Black Doris plums, the Roxburgh Red apricots like those from the family orchard, preserved in an electric Vacola water bath. As a teenager, Matt used to eat a whole jar for afternoon tea. There was homemade jam and chutney too, and tomato sauce in thick glass bottles with swing lids.

The day after I wrote the word 'Vacola', having not thought of it for 30 years, I met a friend at a local café. On the wall was a 1950s poster of a smiling housewife in a gingham apron and high heels, advertising a Vacola juice extractor. On the table beside her were a pile of veges and those sauce bottles from my childhood. At that moment I felt aligned with the universe.

MUM'S PERSONAL RECIPE book was her bible. Lined and bound with a hard crimson cover, it was a social as well as culinary record, beginning with 'Faggots' (chopped liver and onion balls, wrapped in bacon) and directions for making soap, and ending with shrimp cocktail and mushroom salad. By the time I was a teenager, the cookbook was dog-eared and stained, bulging with yellowed clippings sellotaped alongside hundreds of recipes in Mum's looping handwriting.

I decided to surprise Mum and rewrite it in a practical ring-binder with a red plastic cover. Whenever she went out, I reproduced each entry in my childish, backward-leaning script. It took many hours. I gave it to her for her birthday. She thanked me and put it on the shelf. She never took it down. Once I asked her why. She said it didn't feel right. She wasn't sentimental about our gifts: her sense of the aesthetic overrode any desire to please us. I knew what she meant. The new cookbook lacked the character, the authority, the history of the original. I never used it either.

Unlike her other domestic skills, Mum's love of cooking rubbed off on me, although I don't remember learning at her side. In the kitchen as elsewhere, she adopted a laissez-faire approach. If you wanted to bake a cake or a batch of biscuits on a Saturday afternoon, she'd be off out into the garden, her parting words, 'You can make what you like as long as you clean up.' (This injunction failed dismally in my case, Pat laments.)

As dusk approached, she'd return, wash the dirt off her hands and throw two legs of lamb in the oven to feed eight of us and any extras. Everyone was welcome, second helpings the norm, dessert guaranteed.

In the early days, Pat found our dinner table daunting: the late meals, the bounty provided by Mum, the conversation led by Dad. Food went on the table in his house the minute his father walked in from the freezing works, and everyone bolted it down in case they missed out. Haunted by our eating rituals, he sent me an aerogramme during his OE in South America on which he'd drawn a plate surrounded by cutlery, with the question, 'Where does the fork go?'

Our culinary preoccupation and generally lean physiques still bemuse Pat. 'I've never seen a family that talks so much about food and eats so little of it,' he says. I prefer my father's explanation that *you can't fatten a thoroughbred*. Dad had an adage for every occasion: *the best things come in small packages*, to boost my five-foot-two-and-a-half-inch morale; *stand not upon the order of thy going but be gone*, usually after he'd kept us talking at the door for half an hour.

All things in moderation was another of his favourites, one that Mum seemed to have forgotten. All over town we'd had to put up 'red flags' asking people to take her phone calls, agree to her demands and then contact us. At the Honda service centre when she booked in the car she no longer owned. At Meticulous Maids when she cancelled her monthly house-cleaning service, or doubled it, or changed the day. At the dentist, the plumber, the lawyer, the electrician, the bank, the post office, Work and Income. In spite of my reservations about therapeutic fibbing, we were schooling half of Wellington in the dark art, to maintain Planet Rosaleen. And we, like six little moons, were spinning ever faster in her gravitational field.

CHAPTER FOURTEEN

———

HAIR CUTS

MUM HAD BEEN going to David's hair salon in Wadestown once a week since 1965, when our family shifted into the suburb. From Newtown, she continued to drive across the city every Thursday to let him wash and style her fine, straight hair into a bouffant, add colour when needed, then put her under a dryer with a cup of tea, her head covered with rollers.

I read about a hairdresser who had three customers pass away under the hairdryer; she took it as a compliment that they'd felt relaxed enough to do so. That could have been Mum. In David she found a kindred spirit. The hour and a half she spent with him was her one concession to being pampered. He'd done her hair when her mother died, when her husband got sick, when her kids left home, for weddings and birthdays, Christmas and Easter, and just so she could face the world. The appointment had always been important to her. But now it was the high point of her week.

Until the Thursday that Kate discovered Mum had made an appointment with Ginny's hairdresser, Amadeus, in Newtown, for the same time as her appointment with David. Mum said he'd rung to say he couldn't fit her in any more and, while she was very put out after all these years, there were advantages in going somewhere local. This was true. Since Mum had lost her licence, it was a hassle to get her to David's. But it was a fixed point in her unravelling life. We all agreed it was sacrosanct.

Kate cancelled the Amadeus appointment and drove Mum to David's. The following Thursday, she arrived at Colville Street to take her again and found: 'Door locked, alarm on, no one home . . . Yellow Pages open to taxis . . . Where could she have gone? Wait for 1/2 hour. Have a brainwave. Call Amadeus. Yes, Mrs Desmond is here. Ask them to hang on to her until I get there. Call David — explain — very understanding. Pick up a very glum Mum who's furious she's sat in a cold salon with an absolute beginner — who's given her . . . curls! (I think they're kind of cute).'

'Let's just say we all have bad hair days,' Rose replied. But the days turned to weeks. In spite of the cold and the curls, Mum kept phoning Amadeus, adamant David was too busy to see her. A new setting had taken hold in her mind. We asked Amadeus to pretend to accept a booking if Mum rang, and let us know. But when Mum used her taxi chits to turn up without an appointment, and demanded service, they could hardly refuse.

We were used to Mum sabotaging arrangements she didn't like. But this was different. David was one of her favourite people. It didn't make sense for her to cut him out of her life. Unless acting normally around those who knew her well had got too hard; unless it was easier to deal with strangers. Whatever the reason, Mum closed the door on David and never re-opened it. A line had been crossed. Slowly she'd whittled down her friends; he can take credit for being the last to go. Now she just wanted us. For everything.

If emails were the barometer of our emotional temperature, September 2006 was the hottest month on record: 28. Before the month was out, Rose, Mum's staunchest advocate, emailed, 'It seems to me that all this is pointing towards Mum getting closer and closer to having to leave her home. Did I say that?!!' Mum's slow decline had ruled out her moving in with Rose and Mike and they were selling their Miramar house. When we called a family meeting, Kate put out a plea for some social time as well: it seemed we only ever met to talk about one thing.

Before we could get together, Megan and Rome found Mum in her chair at Colville Street, doubled over in pain. She'd fallen in the kitchen, she said. No bones broken, but she could hardly walk. We set up a 24-hour roster. At three in the morning, Rose woke to find Mum outside smoking a cigarette. The next afternoon, Matt found her clinging to the bannister at the bottom of the stairs, unable to move. He helped her back to bed where she took two sleeping pills, saying she needed a good sleep because her back was very sore.

In the 15 minutes between Matt leaving and my getting there, Ginny phoned Mum, who told her she was lying on the floor. By the time I arrived, she was bent over the bathroom basin, trying to brush her teeth. Her speech was slurred. As I tucked her into bed, she fixed me with a boozy grin and breathed nicotine fumes over me. A whiff of the glass of 'water' on her bedside table confirmed it was gin.

Mum's GP told us off the record that the quickest way to have Mum's needs reassessed was to get her admitted to Wellington Hospital. She warned it wouldn't be easy. We took it in turns to sit with Mum propped up in a wheelchair in the emergency department waiting room while a procession of the lame and the sick were given higher priority.

When she hadn't been seen by evening, we took her back to Colville Street, stayed with her overnight, then returned next morning. Heartless as it felt to deliver her up like a sacrificial lamb, none of us buckled. Carol from Alzheimers Wellington had said the right time for someone to move out of their house was when the family couldn't cope any more. That time had come.

Towards the end of the second day, Mum was seen by a doctor

and given a bed in a four-person cubicle. The health system took over: a CT scan, occupational therapy assessment, visits from the physiotherapist, dietician and chaplain. Family made a fuss of her. My son Jackson, working in the hospital pharmacy to fund his science degree, put his head round the curtain and they had a great talk, he said. Next day, they had another great talk: the same one.

Mum, who'd always preferred solitude, lapped up the attention and the buzz of the surgical ward. As a doctor's wife, she found the medical world familiar and reassuring. In hospital she was a sick person, not someone losing her mind. The respite was short-lived. Within a couple of days, she was dressing herself and walking well, although she wandered at night. Tests aside, she didn't need further treatment. As soon as the hospital assessed her level of care, we were told, she'd be discharged at a day or two's notice. If we hadn't found somewhere for her to go, they would.

Rose and Kate met with hospital staff, who accepted that Mum couldn't live at home any more. The care coordinator said she didn't think Mum was ready for a rest home. She wanted her to trial a one-room studio in a Wellington retirement village. There was a vacancy two doors down from Mum's old friend Lorna who also had dementia and had apparently settled in well.

THE RETIREMENT VILLAGE was on the other side of town from Rose, Ginny, me and that beacon of light, the Chelsea Club. But it was close to Kate, and the only similar accommodation near the rest of us had a six-month waiting list. My sisters asked the professionals to break the news to Mum. 'There was one flash of anger and a few tears ("I'll have to leave my mother's things") but overall Mum was very accepting,' Kate emailed. 'Not only of the six-week recuperation but also of the possibility of it being a longer-term option.'

The move was scheduled for the following Monday. Emails flew back and forth about signing the paperwork, organising Mum's medication and clothes, choosing furnishings for her studio, letting relatives know. Everyone agreed it would be too unsettling for Mum to go back to Colville Street first. Kate volunteered to set up the studio with Ginny the day before. But no one offered to pick Mum up from the hospital and deliver her to her new lodgings.

For me, the timing was terrible. I had three weeks to hand in my 100,000-word university thesis, at about the same time as my second grandchild was due. But it was more than that. I couldn't be the bad daughter one more time. I couldn't withstand Mum's fury, her tears, her cold shoulder. Worst of all, I couldn't witness her defeat.

Sobbing, I phoned Liz. Everyone expected me to move Mum into the village, I said, perhaps wrongly. I couldn't do it; I didn't even know if I could visit her there for a while. Liz listened till I stopped crying, promised to talk to the others, and offered to come down from Hastings to move Mum herself if necessary.

Rose, convalescing after an operation, said it wasn't fair for me to bow out; there weren't enough of us as it was. I knew everyone was worn out. I knew everyone was reeling from the guilt of becoming one of those families 'who put a parent into care'. I knew it couldn't be me.

Ginny and Kate, bless them, picked Mum up from hospital and took her to the retirement village. That night Kate emailed to say it had gone well. 'At 8 p.m. I called the night nurse to see how Mum had settled. She said she'd had a lovely afternoon with Lorna, had just been given her Triazolam, and said she looked very cozy in bed with her little hat on. What hat, you ask? — as did I. Not sure, but think she may have gone to bed wearing a shower cap!'

There was one silver lining. My siblings agreed that Megan and Rome could move into Colville Street until we decided what to do with the house. They'd have their own place, close to Pat and me, to bring their second baby home.

CHAPTER FIFTEEN

PARTY OVER

I NEED MY HOUSE KEYS TO PICK UP SOME CLOTHES
(SEEING AS PIP HAS BOOKED ME IN FOR 8 WEEKS)
— I WILL NOT STAY 8 WEEKS. I'D GO BANANAS — &
REGISTRAR TOLD ME THIS A.M. I DO NOT HAVE TO STAY
8 WEEKS. SURGEON WILL BE IN NEXT WEEK AND GIVE
ME AN IDEA ABOUT DISCHARGE. (HE MIGHT WANT TO
LOOK AT SUITABILITY OF HOUSE) — I LEFT IT CLEAN
AND TIDY.

I AM FURIOUS, FRUSTRATED AND UPSET. VERY. PHONE I
ORDERED HAD BEEN RETURNED. RECEPTION SAID ONE
OF MY DAUGHTERS CANCELLED IT — AS I DIDN'T NEED
IT. (And described her!! So I know who it was.) OWN UP. I
DON'T NEED ALL THIS. I DO NEED CLEAN CLOTHES.

I wouldn't recommend ANYONE TO COME HERE. SERVICE
TERRIBLE — FOOD AWFUL (standard deteriorated
since arrived) considering COST (NICE VIEW FROM MY

WINDOW!) ALL AT MY TABLE (5 of us) agree about food and service — they have already complained to Dining Room Supervisor to no avail. Once you have signed in, you are helpless. My 'caregiver' is downright rude — is she menopausal???

I AM FED UP AND CROSS. Have phoned Reception but they have no spare remotes. TV doesn't work without remote. Ginny took Remote — as wanted to buy one like mine. SO AT 7 p.m. there's nothing to do but go to bed.

PHONE RECEPTION re Hair Appointment. Where is RECEPTION ???? (Upstairs.)

I'D WALK OUT EXCEPT I'M TOLD SECURITY AT FRONT DOOR DEMAND TO SEE DISCHARGE FORM. BEEN HERE ? WEEKS AND SEEN NO ONE EXCEPT THE CLEANER. AM COMPLETELY FED UP. NO WAY I'M STAYING HERE 8 WEEKS.

I AM IN THE WRONG PLACE — I'VE SAID BEFORE AND YOU IGNORE ME. WHY??? I CAN'T BELIEVE MY FAMILY WHO'VE BEEN SO SPECIAL TO ME ARE DOING THIS. GUESS I'VE PASSED MY USEFUL DATE. I'VE GONE DOWN TO PATIENTS LOUNGE (ONCE) — SO DEPRESSING. HAVING BEEN TOLD THIS WAS FOR ONE WEEK — I HAVEN'T ENOUGH CLOTHES AND CAN'T GO HOME TO GET MORE. SOME NIGHTS I JUST CRY.

Mum recorded her distress in handwritten notes taped to the outside of her door and strewn around her studio. Angry, sad, outrageous, astute, pleading, they tugged at our hearts and threatened our resolve. When we went to see her, she'd often still be in her dressing gown, emptying her kitchen cupboards, packing her personal belongings into a bag. She hated having no landline, her link to the outside world. We were just as dismayed about the three-week wait to get one installed but nothing would convince her we hadn't cut it off deliberately.

People suggested we stop visiting her for a while to give her a chance to settle in. But we didn't want to abandon her to strangers and couldn't check on her without a phone. After several weeks she insisted that Pat, the only one who hadn't been to see her, was the only one who had. He used this as ammunition in the long-running contest for favourite son-in-law. Our husbands had always wooed Mum shamelessly. While Pat was tempting her with a pot of new spuds from his garden, Rose's husband Mike would be whispering in her ear, 'That's small potatoes, Rosaleen. How about a glass of my fine chardonnay?'

Mum was in no mood to be kidded now. 'You might as well all live on the other side of the world, the amount I see you,' she'd protest. From her point of view, it was true. She didn't know how fast time passed, couldn't fill the hours with reading and crossword puzzles. Her memory of us disappeared with our departing backs.

In those early days we didn't take her out of the village for fear it would be too hard to take her back. But when Rose celebrated her fiftieth birthday at Waikanae, we decided that a taste of the outside world couldn't make Mum more miserable than she already was.

Pat and I and Matt's wife, Hang, went to pick her up and found her sitting on her bed, staring at the door. Grudgingly she changed out of her fleecy jacket with a toothpaste dribble down the front, ran a red lipstick across her lips and put a comb through her hair. It looked softer and more natural since she'd stopped having it dyed and permed at David's.

On the hour's drive up the coast, Mum's melancholy lifted. She exclaimed over the toetoe and yellow broom brightening up the highway, the cluster of caravans for sale at Mana, the first glimpse of Kāpiti Island sprawled along the horizon, the Paraparaumu boat shop where Dad had bought the heavy wooden dinghy he named Pippi (after the shellfish, he said, but my bursting 10-year-old heart knew better). 'It's so good to be out,' she kept saying, as if she were on parole.

Mum had always been an asset on a road trip: happy to sit in the back, never car sick or irritable, stepping out at the destination looking as fresh as when she'd set off. After she'd been caring for Dad for too long, we packed her off to London for a month to stay with Kate and her husband Andy. She was an ideal travelling companion, cooperative, punctual and well organised. She'd happily go off on a bus tour by herself, always found somewhere to get her hair done, and continued to order a cooked breakfast and substantial pub lunch long after others had cried off them.

After that first trip on her own, Mum would go anywhere in the world to see her children: Vancouver, Kuwait, Hanoi. She was over 70 when she made her last trip to Bangkok to mark the birth of her youngest grandchild, Sarah, by which time she was practically a regular at the Sheraton jazz club. Her one concession as she got older was to request a wheelchair to get on and off the plane and deal with her luggage: she could swallow her pride when it suited her.

AT ROSE AND Mike's the rain came down and everyone crammed into their beach house. Every time I looked, Mum was surrounded by well-wishers. She'd been the queen of conversation and her social cues were still sharp. Unless they knew better, or stayed to talk a while, her fans would never guess how hard her brain was working.

I heard someone ask her about the retirement village and edged closer.

'There's nothing wrong with it,' she said to my astonishment. She paused: 'It *is* claustrophobic.' This was true. If she stayed, she'd need a bigger studio than the one she was trialling. She embarked on a story about five men who always sat by themselves in the communal dining room. Where were their wives, Mum had asked a staff member? 'Glad to get rid of the old boys,' the staff member replied. Mum chortled at the thought of it, and others joined in.

Rose's friend arrived with his mother who also had vascular dementia. He'd taken her to live with him and she seemed cheerful and resigned to her new circumstances. Guilt reared up in me that we hadn't opened our homes to Mum. I reminded myself that she seemed cheerful and resigned at that moment too.

After the speeches and toasts, Ginny and Kate brought out a giant chocolate cake ablaze with candles. When we were kids, Mum always made us a cake for our birthdays. With her grandkids, she went a step further, creating works of art — a castle, a swimming pool, a soccer field, a witch — well beyond my own skill and patience.

Every second year, we'd been allowed a party. But at the bottom of the invitations, Mum always wrote, 'No presents, please', no matter how much we begged her not to. She didn't want other mothers going to the trouble and expense, she'd say — although we took presents to their kids' parties, and Mum had a drawer in her bedroom where she kept a supply of gifts for every occasion.

The 'no presents' rule didn't apply to her and Dad. For Christmas and birthdays, he'd give us books, she more worldly treasures. My favourite was the pale blue shoulder bag she bought me when I turned 11, the chic-est thing I'd ever owned. It must have been a party year because Dad took me and my friends to see *It's a Mad, Mad, Mad, Mad World* on the new wide screen at the Cinerama Theatre in Courtenay Place. We came home to the smell of schnitzel and homemade chips, orange juice and lemonade in red stemmed glasses, a cake with a ruffle around it.

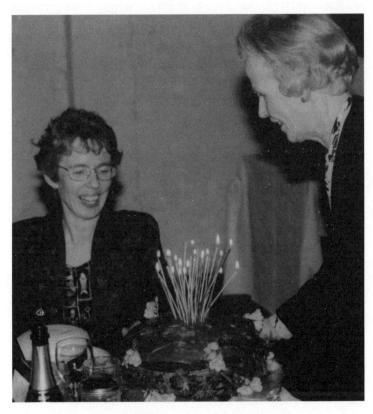

Mum was still baking me her special chocolate
cake when I turned 40 in August 1995.

When we tried to give Mum a blow-by-blow description of the movie, she'd have said, 'Don't tell me, I might want to go and see it,' as she always did. It wasn't till the next morning I realised I'd left the blue bag in the cinema. She made me phone about it but it was gone. I still feel a pang, as if my whole life might have been more glamorous if I'd managed to hang on to it for more than 24 hours.

In those years, Mum and Dad often threw parties themselves, classy affairs with men in dinner suits and women in evening dress. For Mum, there'd be days of food preparation, flower arranging and housework leading up to them. We kids would be roped in on the night to serve drinks and nibbles and clean up the kitchen. It was fun as long as some well-meaning or tipsy adult didn't bail me up: unlike Mum, I was hopeless at small talk.

After Dad got sick, their own parties stopped, although they still let us have them from time to time. Being so close in age to Matt and Liz became a bonus in my teenage years when Mum and Dad provided not just food for scores of their friends but also alcohol, on the optimistic premise the party-goers wouldn't top it up. I don't remember there being gate-crashers or trouble. I do remember the first big party I hosted myself when I left college. Mum made me a long blue smock dress with tiny pink flowers and puffed sleeves, and I floated around all night in bare feet, feeling like a hippie.

At Rose's fiftieth, the guitars came out and the noise went up a notch. Mum showed no signs of flagging. Around nine, we finally said our goodbyes. By the time we'd rejoined the highway, she'd forgotten she'd been at a party and sat silently in the back seat with Hang as we drove through the night. Her daughter-in-law, far from her own mother in Vietnam, loved her with a quiet resolve; she even called her 'Mum'.

WHEN WE PULLED into the retirement village, Mum said nothing. I was grateful not to be doing this alone: she always behaved better when other people were around. Pat dropped us at the entrance and went to park the car. At the carers' station, a staff member gave Mum a sleeping pill and watched her take it with a glass of water. Then Hang and I walked her past the communal lounge, through the heavy swing doors, down the long, narrow corridor studded left and right with identical, numbered entrances to the studios. What a leveller old age was, I thought. No matter how eventful or high-powered, no matter how full of friends and family and possessions, the lives behind each door were all ending the same way: alone in a single bed in a small room in an institution.

Somehow Mum recognised the number on her own door. It wasn't locked, making her seem childlike and vulnerable. But staff had to be able to get in, I told myself, and a key was just another thing to lose. Inside, she took off her coat, picked up a note in her handwriting and started to read: 'Walking stick. Anybody know where it is? Who has my grey cardigan, my handbag and my mirror?'

A wave of tiredness hit me. I put out my hand. 'We're not doing this now, Mum,' I said. To my surprise, she gave me the note. I found her pyjamas, turned back her sheets and dithered until it became clear she wouldn't get into bed in front of us.

On the way out, we passed a man and two women sitting in front of the gas fire in the lounge. I stopped to ask where I could find the staff member who was no longer at reception. I wanted her to check on Mum; I was worried the sleeping pill might take effect before she made it into bed.

The younger of the two women, about my age, was bent over a needlepoint canvas. She said the studio area was classified as independent living and staff went off duty at ten. A staff member would come over from the rest home if a resident rang the bell beside their bed. But if they rang it too often, they'd be transferred to the rest home. This was something new to worry about: how Mum would find the bell, if she'd think to ring it, how she'd stop once she started.

The woman told me she and her husband weren't visitors as I'd assumed. When her mother bought an apartment at the village, they'd bought one too. I didn't dare ask her how it was working out.

I asked Pat and Hang to wait in the car while I went back to check on Mum. Outside her studio door, I heard water running. I waited a minute, knocked and went in.

She was sitting with one foot on the bed, peeling off her stockings. She looked up. 'What are you doing here?' she asked, more weary than startled.

'I just wanted to make sure you're all right.'

She fumbled with the buttons on her cardigan. 'Yes, I'm all right.'

I longed to rush over, scoop her into my arms and take her with me. Instead, I stood in the middle of the room, not knowing what to do.

She made a shooing motion with her hands. 'You've got to go now, you've got work tomorrow.'

I turned away so she couldn't see my tears. 'Goodnight, Mum.'

'Goodnight.'

In the empty corridor, I rested my forehead against her door. From the other side came muffled noises like those of a small animal building its nest. My heart felt like it would break. This knowing mother was wiser than me, and more courageous. *You can't help me,* she was saying. *I have to do this thing alone.*

CHAPTER SIXTEEN

BOARDING SCHOOL BLUES

TWO DOZEN WOMEN were sitting in the communal lounge at the retirement village. They had a well-to-do, if slightly dishevelled, air; the one brown face stood out. There was no sign of the five men whose wives were glad to be rid of them. I was relieved to see Mum among them, not moping in her studio.

'You're late,' she said. She laughed when my eyebrows went up — I hadn't told her I was coming — and patted the empty seat beside her.

A staff member offered us tea and biscuits from a trolley. I turned to the woman next to me and asked how long she'd lived there, part of the informal resident satisfaction survey I was conducting. 'Three weeks,' she said, although I knew better than to take her at her word.

'How are you finding it?'

'Terrible,' she said. 'Worst decision I made in my life. Now it's too late to go back.'

Across the room, I caught the eye of Mum's old friend, Lorna. She returned my wave. I wondered if she recognised me or was just responding to a friendly face. Before Mum moved into the village, I'd contacted her daughter, Catherine. We'd been best friends at school, both middle children from big families with fathers who were doctors and mothers who did everything on the home front. (Actually our family was only middle-sized in Catholic terms; you had to have at least eight kids, as hers did, to qualify as big.)

Catherine told me Lorna was happy at the village. Her mother had a sunny disposition and that hadn't changed, she said, which made me wince about Mum's deep-seated distress.

Their home had been both more easy-going and more conservative than ours. When I stayed the night, Lorna let us have midnight feasts and abandoned the housework to listen to our piano duets. But Catherine's father led the family in five decades of the Rosary — not just one, like Dad — rattling them off so fast that, kneeling in front of a chair, I'd have to push my face into the cushion to stifle my giggles.

Lorna had had her own share of sorrow, losing not only her husband but two sons, one when he was only 20. Thinking of Sally Magnusson's theory of supressed grief, I wonder how she'd mourned them — how any parent successfully mourns the death of a child.

'I should go over and say hello,' I said to Mum.

Mum looked doubtful. 'She's very deaf, you know.' She changed the subject. 'There's a management committee meeting next week. They've put out a suggestion box and I've recommended that all staff should wear name tags.' We glanced around the room. All the staff were wearing name tags. 'Oh, look,' she said, 'they've implemented it already.'

A woman approached us, looking flustered. She'd missed the tea service so I gave her my chair, went over to the trolley and brought her back a cup. A minute later, I saw her up at the trolley trying to lift the heavy teapot herself.

'You get all sorts in here,' sniffed the woman who'd told me the place was terrible.

'She's just a bit forgetful,' I said, feeling oddly protective.

'Like me,' said Mum who usually denied the slightest suggestion of memory loss.

I retrieved the flustered woman and pointed out her cup of tea, only to see her head back to the trolley almost at once, at the mercy of some cruel impulse that made her spring up like a jack-in-the-box every time she sat down.

As Mum and I made our way to her studio, we were stopped by a tall woman in a twin set and pearls. In the interests of my survey, I asked her if she liked the village.

'Happy as a sand boy,' she boomed. 'I don't take it too seriously. Plenty of practice. I went to boarding school.'

'That's what I thought on the first day,' Mum said. 'Just like boarding school.'

'Only the food's better,' I suggested.

'And you're allowed to talk on the stairs,' Mum said.

At this, she and the woman roared with laughter like old war buddies. The stairs weren't the only place where boarders were forbidden to speak at St Dominic's College in the 1940s. There was no talking in the dormitory, the bathroom or the study hall either. Or at meals, where a nun read to the girls — except on Saturdays at breakfast when they were allowed to talk, as long as it was in French. 'You could go for twenty-four hours without speaking, more or less,' Mum said. For teenage girls, it sounded like the definition of torture.

In *Windows on a Women's World*, a history of the New Zealand Dominican sisters, author Susannah Grant says life in the boarding school was modelled on life in the convent. 'The regulations were strict. Each morning pupils were woken by a bell (at 5.55 a.m. in summer and 6.30 a.m. in winter). The dormitory sister went around each bed sprinkling holy water. While the girls dressed she led them in their morning prayers. Before the girls left for class they presented brushes, combs and fingers for inspection . . . Noisiness, lateness and personal untidiness were not tolerated . . . When they moved about within the school, the girls walked silently in assigned pairs.'

I began to understand why Mum had been so kind to my boarder friends at college who spent innumerable Sundays at our house. As their curfew approached, she could always be counted on to ring the boarding mistress to explain why they needed to stay on for tea. Sundays at St Dom's were particularly deadly, she told me. 'Especially Sunday afternoons because you weren't allowed to play tennis or any sport or do anything active. You weren't allowed to knit or sew or embroider or anything like that. So you were pretty hard-stretched, weren't you?'

Overcome with boredom one such afternoon, Mum and a friend — wearing their 'costumes', the black skirt and jacket reserved for Sundays — played hooky to buy biscuits from the dairy. 'We got back and everything was fine and then we were called to the Mistress of Boarders' office,' Mum said. 'And one of those sneaky nuns had been watching us from those big, high windows in the convent. She'd seen us slip out, she'd seen us come back.' Their monthly Sunday leave was cancelled. 'We had to stay there, the only two people in that great, big rattling place. And she reported it to our parents, who thought it was hilarious. You can imagine, it was so humiliating when she told your parents what you'd done. It was a joke in the family for ages.'

Mum offered this as her worst moment at college: what a good girl she must have been. She also said, 'It's funny. In spite of all the discipline that was absolutely absurd, we weren't unhappy. We were OK.'

After coming across the term 'boarding school syndrome' coined by British psychotherapist Dr Joy Schaverien, I wondered if this was true. Children can be left with lifelong scars when they have to shut down their emotions to cope with the institutional demands of boarding school and the early rupture of family life, Schaverien says. While younger children are worst affected, Mum's years at St Dom's taught her to supress her emotions too. Quoting from School Customs enforced until the early 1960s, Susannah Grant says, 'Sisters were expected to monitor the girls during recreation hours, guard against unduly intimate relationships and guide conversation away from dangerous topics such as balls, theatres, dress, young gentlemen, family arrangements, criticism whether of school rules, or of the nuns or of each other.'

Certainly Mum's move into the retirement village triggered an antipathy towards authority that seemed to stem from her college days. One of the first new things she learned to do was to write her name in the day book at reception when she went out and tick it off when she came back. As time went on, the ticks got larger, sometimes covering a whole page, not necessarily the one with her name on it. Sometimes she formed the tick with a flourish, as if to confirm her existence. More often, the gesture was laced with anger: *I, Rosaleen Desmond, obey the rules because I have to.*

Mum didn't always obey the rules. A carer bailed me up to say my mother was a very determined woman. I felt the same surge of pride as when Barb, the Chelsea Club manager, had said she was strong, although this time it wasn't meant as a compliment. Mum had refused to let the carer make her bed. 'I don't need to because my daughter is coming to take me home for good,' she'd shouted.

I could understand why. She'd have hated the intrusion into her private space. And she was used to making her own bed, but now she couldn't because it was pushed against the wall, the only place it would fit in the small room.

Moving into the village made Mum safer, but it erased most of her control over her life and almost all the activities that had occupied her day. From the moment her breakfast arrived at 7.30 a.m., she was waited on, with no opportunity to help or contribute. She couldn't even have a bath, her morning ritual for as long as I could remember. Instead, she was expected to let a stranger help her shower three mornings a week. She quickly became victim to the 'Three Plagues' of nursing homes identified by American surgeon Atul Gawande in his thought-provoking book *Being Mortal*: helplessness, boredom and loneliness.

Seeing Mum succumb was sadder than seeing her get angry. She stopped doing even the things she was capable of. We'd find her clothes draped over the furniture or lying on the floor. This would have been unthinkable to the old house-proud mother whose folded washing looked like it had been ironed. We wondered whether she'd forgotten where the clothes went or just didn't care.

'She probably doesn't think the wardrobe's hers,' suggested the manager of a rest home I was visiting as we canvassed other options. The manager was sympathetic about Mum's opposition to showering. Creating conflict was counter-productive, she said. 'So what if someone only showers once a week?' We longed for similar empathy at the retirement village where it seemed to us there was little understanding of, or allowance made for, dementia, although my informal survey had shown it was widespread among studio residents. Instead, those who didn't comply with the rules were treated like naughty children.

I asked the rest home manager what she thought of Mum's retirement village and its parent company. 'They do what they do well,' she said. 'But you mustn't forget, their focus is real estate, ours is health care.' She'd summed up our dilemma. Some of the rest homes we visited, particularly the not-for-profit ones, seemed kinder and more progressive but their facilities were shabby and their residents more physically disabled than Mum. It was hard to imagine her making the transition from her big house to a bedroom the size of a cubicle where she had to share a bathroom with a stranger. Larger rooms with views and en suites had waiting lists. The dementia units were the most depressing of all: residents slumped in chairs, muttering to themselves, pacing circular corridors, jiggling the handles of locked doors. One woman followed us with a fixed look of astonishment, her eyebrows arched, her mouth in a frozen 'O'. Mum couldn't go there, she wasn't like that. *Not yet*, said a voice in my head.

I scurried away, disheartened by how long old people could live and how much care they needed and how hard it was to treat them with dignity. Growing up, I hadn't had much to do with old age. Sometimes we'd visit Dad's two maiden aunts — who lived in the narrow, two-storey family house in Thorndon with a stall for the horse that had pulled his grandfather's hansom cab — and they fed us lemonade and wine biscuits. But Mum's mother Dolly was the only grandparent I knew and we only saw her once or twice a year.

When she became ill in her mid-seventies, Dolly came to stay with us in Wadestown. There was nothing wrong with her mind, I don't think, but one afternoon she emptied her bowels on her way to the bathroom. Liz, 14, and I, a year younger, were the only ones home. I remember fleeing and leaving my big sister to clean her up. After that, the sickly smell of death emanated from the bedroom at the other end of the hall and I was too scared to go near my warm-hearted grandmother who'd made me feel so special.

Grandma died in Calvary Hospital on Ginny's birthday. 'She looks beautiful, so peaceful,' Dad said when he rang with the news. I felt deceived when we were taken to see her. To me, she looked blue and waxy and lifeless, though Rose remembers her as Dad described.

Death was not hidden from us Catholics. In my college days at St Mary's, the word would go round, 'There's a dead nun in the chapel'. We'd head over at lunchtime, bless ourselves with holy water and stare into the open casket in front of the altar, trying to make the link between the dense corpse and our own alive young bodies. Once there were two caskets: bloodless old women, faces framed by veils and wimples.

Such images had no place in the retirement village. The reception area looked like a hotel lobby and there was a huge atrium where my one-year-old grandson tried to catch the goldfish swimming in an open water channel. Atul Gawande says aged-care facilities pitch such features not at prospective residents but at their anxious offspring who mistake glamour for good care.

Later, we'd discover the rest home and hospital rooms were poor cousins to the attractive studios we were being shown. But for now we were seduced by the movies on the big screen in the communal lounge, the onsite hairdresser and library, the downstairs dining room and bar. The studio area didn't have the boiled-cabbage-and-urine smell of some older rest homes. We would learn that it didn't have their heart either.

MUM CELEBRATED HER seventy-seventh birthday 'on the first sunny day we've had in living memory (Mum's & mine at least!)', Kate emailed Matt. Among the guests was our new granddaughter, Avah, three days old. In the same email, Kate said the psycho-geriatrician nurse had called to set up another assessment of Mum. 'We spoke for 30 mins — she was very understanding & supportive. She reminded me that Mum's illness is slowly progressive, she will deteriorate and become more dependent. At the moment Mum's short term memory has gone, but her social graces are still intact. She needs structure & routine.'

Kate was present at the assessment which took the form of a casual chat, she said. The psychiatrist — the same one who'd recommended Mum give up driving — 'appeared to have a pre-formed opinion that Mum was not "competent" (from hospital records, her referral to the studio, staff?). Which she proved as he led her through a discussion on the pros and cons of living at home compared with her studio. "I don't think it would be a good idea at all for me to go back home," she said. "At home I'm on my own and I have all the responsibility." As she left, the nurse whispered to me, "She's in the right place." Which I took to mean the level of care.'

Mum never told *me* it wasn't a good idea for her to go home. Our conversations went more like this:

Mum: 'I've just written you a note. The registrar said I can go home this week. I told him to ring you because you're the one who booked me in.' My attempt to distance myself from the move had failed.

Me: 'It was a family decision, Mum.'

'Why?'

'Because you've lost your memory and you can't look after yourself.'

'What can't I do?'

'You forget to eat.'

'No, I don't.'

'And we're scared you'll fall again.'

'Well, I hate it here.'

'I know it's hard.'

'It's easy for you to say that. You've never been locked up in a little room.'

'I know.'

'It's easy to say "I know". That doesn't do anything.'

'Sorry, Mum, we've looked everywhere and talked to everyone we can. This is the best we can come up with.'

Mum, crying now: 'If I had the guts, I'd throw myself out the window.'

Looking back, I'm appalled at my unskilful handling of these exchanges. I was willing to use the therapeutic fibbing for the little things, but I still thought it was dishonest. I wanted to be straight with Mum. I wanted her to face up to her illness and accept her limitations. I didn't understand that she couldn't.

We shared Mum's reservations about the retirement village. But as her six-week studio trial ticked away and no other clear option emerged, the pressure went on us to buy one. Mum was lucky she could afford the tough financial terms in the complicated contract. On top of a $163,000 'licence to occupy' (more than a decade ago), she'd have to pay almost $400 a week for a care package that included meals (whether or not she ate them), personal laundry (that Kate often did), night visits (if she pushed that bell) and help with showering and medication (should she accept it). When the studio was sold, she'd get back 80 per cent of the purchase price, a negative rate of return almost unheard of for other real estate. Since then, the parent company has increased profit by around 15 per cent, year in, year out — and yet, like its counterparts in New Zealand, it's paid no tax in that time. There's big money being made out of old folk.

But the rest home option would also be costly for Mum. Although she wouldn't have to buy the right to occupy her room, her weekly rate of care would be about twice as high as in a studio. She had too many assets to qualify for government assistance. Over eight years she'd fork out a similar amount either way, with no asset at the end if she went into a rest home.

Not that any of this mattered. Dad had left Mum financially secure and our only consideration was what was best for her. Which 'her', though? The mother with social skills and insight, acutely aware of her surroundings and desperate to be independent, would probably do better in a studio. The confused, angry, vulnerable mother was more likely to get the personal care and attention she needed in a rest home. We decided the first mother was in front by a nose. We weren't sure, though. Rose summed up our misgivings about the retirement village when she emailed: 'Just want us to remember that she probably won't now (or ever) receive the kind of care at the level that we think she really needs, particularly in the longer term. As long as we're OK with that.'

'I do question my reasons for choosing the studio option,' Liz replied. 'Is it because I have found the rest homes to be depressing that I'm against Mum going there? Would she actually not mind the things that would bother me — the lack of privacy, the restricted spaces, the incontinence, the walking frames, etc? Would the caring "ambience" compensate for her? Is it a way of denying her condition that I'm hoping to keep her in the most "normal" surroundings possible? Maybe. I guess my own stuff can't help but get mixed up in it.'

In the end, moving Mum felt more fraught — and the outcome less predictable — than keeping her where she was. If it didn't work out, we comforted ourselves, we'd sell up her studio and move on.

CHAPTER SEVENTEEN

───

A NEW FRIEND

MUM'S UNIT WAS one of the nicest studios in the village, a combined bedroom and living room with an en suite like the others, but bigger than most and with a straight run down the hall to the communal lounge. The window overlooked a pristine bowling green that I never saw in use.

We decided not to tell Mum she'd bought the studio or take her back to Colville Street — where Megan and Rome had moved in with their two small children — until she was more settled. We asked her what furniture she'd like and wrote a list. Next time I looked, she'd added 'DESK' twice (Dad's hefty roll-top), 'BOOK CASE', 'DINING TABLE AND CHAIRS' (the 12 seater), 'COUCH' and 'RUGS'. I wondered where she thought it was all going to go.

Liz organised the paperwork from Hastings. Two cheerful removal men — one missing a front tooth, the other with a bad back — delivered the items in a small truck. Mum shadowed Ginny and me as we covered her single bed with a mohair blanket, stocked the fridge, tucked a small table into the far corner and set up her stereo and TV.

I handed Mum some china cups and saucers wrapped in newspaper and suggested she put them in her mother's oak cabinet. She unwrapped them and handed them back to me, unable to take the next step. But she hadn't lost her eye for décor and was quick to tell us if anything was out of place.

By the time we'd covered the carpet with the big rug from her lounge, the room looked like a mini-Colville Street: tasteful, welcoming, very full. There was even a landline. I called Liz in Hastings to check it was working and handed Mum the phone. 'Hang on a minute,' I heard her say. She turned to me. 'I've got a spare bed, haven't I?'

'Liz will still come and see you,' I said, disconcerted anew by the parallel universe Mum inhabited. There wasn't space for a coat stand, let alone a roommate.

Lorna and another woman turned up. They poked through Mum's cupboards, admired the photos and ornaments along her low bookcase and settled themselves in her comfortable chairs. We made them a cup of tea and left them to their round-and-round musings.

On the way out, I picked up a note Mum had written on the back of the furniture list:

> M.'s daughter, she is a police woman (M. is my table mate)
> tells me what you lot have done to incarcerate me in here
> for 8 WEEKS — MY ADMISSION FORM SAYS 8 DAYS —
> I'VE SEEN IT — when surgeon had told me 8 days for rehab
> — this is a criminal offence and I should report it to the
> police. I won't, but I am VERY upset and unhappy. I HAVE
> TO GET CLOTHES — so somehow have to get home (the
> rule is NO NIGHT CLOTHES in dining room).

Having to name all Mum's belongings reinforced the boarding school association. She sat at my kitchen table writing 'R Desmond' on strips of labels and passing them to me to cut up and iron onto her clothes. It may not have been wise to involve her but it passed the time and the job needed to be done.

Mum's eyes flicked to the clock above the fridge. 'I need to go soon, they're expecting me for lunch,' she said. Much as she hated eating in the dining room, as midday approached she'd begin to fret that she had to be back. The institution already had a hold on her.

Distraction arrived in the form of Megan with four-week-old Avah and 15-month-old Rome. I hoped Mum wouldn't look out the window and see her red Honda parked in the lane. We hadn't told her we'd bought it for Megan. The news that she was living at Colville Street had unleashed enough angry phone calls for Megan to deal with.

I tried to intercept Mum's notes before she saw them:

DEAR MEGAN, I URGENTLY NEED TO GET INTO MY
HOUSE FOR CLOTHES, MAIL (WHAT ARE YOU DOING
ABOUT MY MAIL??) & OTHER NECESSITIES. I HAVE
ALREADY TRIED — BUT DOOR WAS BOLTED — THIS
HAS BECOME URGENT AND ANNOYING. PLEASE PHONE
ME A.S.A.P. IT IS MY HOME, REMEMBER — I WANT TO
CHECK UP — TELL ME WHEN CONVENIENT. GRANDMA.

While I prepared lunch, I sat Mum on the cane couch and handed her the dark-haired baby girl. Her face softened. 'What can I buy for her?' she asked over and over again, the generous great-grandmother restored. It reminded me of what Liz had said after seeing Mum twice in one day, the first time delightful, the second, ghastly: 'She truly is like someone with multiple personalities, she even looked physically different.'

As Mum cleared the dishes off the table, she scraped chicken bones and scraps into the children's nappy bag. It was the first

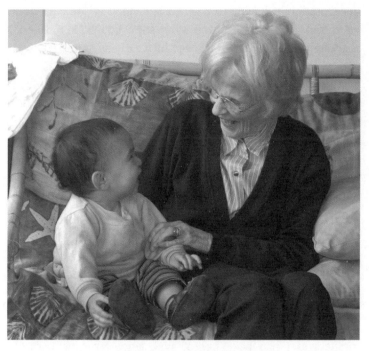

Mum and Rome enjoy a joke, 2006.

really strange thing I'd seen her do, although the hubbub of little ones was enough to addle anyone's brain.

Next morning Rose called in on her way to work to pick up Mum's clothes. I hadn't finished ironing the labels and sensed her irritation at having to wait. As she stood at the back door, we talked about when to tell Mum she'd bought her studio. I suggested we take our time. Rose said we'd rushed into buying it and now I wanted to go slowly.

All I heard was that everything was my fault, just as Mum alleged. Lights danced in front of my eyes and my head felt as if it would burst. From a long way away, I heard myself scream, 'You're not the only one who loves our mother, we're all trying to do our best.' I didn't care that my voice rang across the neighbourhood like the *whoop-whoop* of the gibbon in the zoo at the bottom of our street.

Rose stood stony-faced until my rage burnt itself out, then doused the embers with quiet, deadly words of her own before leaving me to sob down the phone again at Liz.

When I'd calmed down, I texted Rose an apology. She texted back, more conciliatory than I deserved. We never talked about it again, but afterwards we were careful with each other, as you are with someone who's in shock.

She and I had been out of sync since Mum got sick. In our childhood twosomes, Pip'n'Rose was a single word, like Matt'n'Liz and Gin'n'Kate. We even looked the same: round faces, straight fringes, those matching dresses. Our closeness as sisters was matched only by our rivalry as siblings. When Rose started smoking cigarettes, I did too, and was left fighting my addiction long after she'd kicked hers. When I set off down the driveway on my wedding day, she called me back. 'Oh, Rose, you're on your own now,' Dad said, and everyone laughed.

In later years Mum took to calling us 'the pouter pigeons'. The description was uncomfortably apt: if we weren't cooing over each other, we were flapping in righteous indignation.

When I started writing this book, I thought it was about dementia. But after reading American writer Vivian Gornick's book *The Situation and The Story: The Art of Personal Narrative,* I changed my mind. 'Every work of literature has both a situation and a story,' Gornick says. 'The situation is the context or circumstance, sometimes the plot; the story is the emotional experience that preoccupies the writer: the insight, the wisdom, the thing one has come to say.'

Using this definition, dementia's just the situation, the backdrop to the real drama. The story's something else entirely. Something about finding my mother, or at least looking for her. Something about family dynamics too: where they come from, the way they shape us, how they reveal themselves in a crisis.

THE PROSPECT OF spending her first Christmas at the retirement village terrified Mum. 'It seems to have a lot to do with the fact that she believes most others will go and the place will be very sad and empty,' Rose emailed after receiving a string of distressed phone calls. 'She spoke of how lonely she is in there and how hard the weekends are because many go home. She told me she feels very abandoned and isolated. And very confined. She is angry with us; angry that she can't go back to her house. Altogether sad and angry.'

A small part of me was pleased that Rose had to field such phone calls too. Mum didn't know the activities programme would stop for two weeks and there'd be fewer staff and less structure at the village than usual. But she knew Christmas was about family and as far as she was concerned, hers had deserted her.

At this time of year in the past, she'd have been making a wreath of dried flowers for her front door, decorating her tree, setting up the nativity scene in the fireplace, glazing the ham, wrapping mini-Christmas cakes in red and green cellophane to give away, putting $20 notes in envelopes for her grandchildren. Instead the days stretched ahead of her, aimless and unproductive.

I brought her home to help me make Christmas mince pies. After lining the patty tins with circles of her decadent cream cheese pastry, I sat her at the table with a bowl of fruit mince. She spooned it into the cases, sealed the lids and pricked them with a fork as expertly as she'd done in her own kitchen for half a century. It was sad to think in her unfamiliar studio she couldn't figure out how to make a cup of tea.

Driving her back to the village (to this day, I can't call it her 'home'), Mum told me Lorna had bought a small house and was going to move it onto the section beside her daughter, Catherine, and rent out her studio. Implausible as this sounded, the message was clear: good children didn't abandon their parents to the care of strangers; they built granny flats next door for them.

I tried to distract Mum. I commiserated about having to leave Colville Street. I talked about the family barbecue we'd be having on Christmas Eve. I said Avah would be smiling by then.

Mum's voice got louder and more reproachful.

Finally I ran out of patience. 'Mum, Lorna might think she's leaving her studio, but she's not going anywhere,' I said. This had nothing to do with allaying Mum's fears, everything to do with convincing her that Catherine wasn't better, kinder, more up to the task of looking after her mother than I was.

'Just like I think I am?' Mum whispered.

'Yes,' I whispered back, patting her knee. There was no joy in the victory.

The rest of the trip passed in silence. But as the sprawling village loomed, Mum became agitated again. 'Are we there already?' she said. 'Oh God, we're nearly there.'

I parked the car, opened the passenger door and helped her out. Clutching my arm, she shuffled towards the entrance as if the breeze was a force nine hurricane. In the lounge, *Gone With the*

Wind was showing on the big screen, the volume uncomfortably high. I suggested we stop and watch it; once she was absorbed, I'd make my getaway.

Mum gave a few people a polite nod as I steered her past six or seven rows of curious eyes towards two empty chairs at the back. 'Watch!' she said, over her shoulder. 'Every head will be turning to see what we're up to.'

Only it can't have been six or seven rows, I realised when I returned to the village 10 years later. There were only three rows of chairs in front of the TV, and no room for any more between the carers' station and the fireplace. The reception area also seemed half the size. I asked a staff member if the layout had changed. No, she said, it had always been like that.

'You were dwarfed by the institution when your mother was living there,' a friend observed. I realised she was right. Mum was not the only one intimidated by her new surroundings. They had the same effect on me.

WE INCLUDED MUM in our Christmas festivities and outings over the summer break as often as our depleted numbers allowed. We did our best to make her studio comfortable too. Ginny and her husband, Gabe, took her shopping for a new armchair. She was keen to have a La-Z-Boy, Ginny emailed, 'but is not able to operate the footrest so it has to be out of the question'.

But none of us brought Mum home to stay — not even after an outbreak of norovirus at the village. Now, I find this hard to believe. A severe stomach bug could have been the end of our 41-kilogram mother. In our defence, she'd only been there for two months: another move would have thrown her and most other residents stayed put as well. The truth is, we were exhausted. But some people do better. Some heroic wives and husbands, partners, sons and daughters find the patience and compassion to live with a loved one who has dementia, not just for a few days but for years. I am in awe of them.

Mum didn't get gastroenteritis over Christmas. She made a new friend, her first in years. Lesla — another Catholic matron with vascular dementia — had been a career woman who wore her past lightly. Lack of visitors didn't seem to bother her; nor did her spartan studio, such a contrast to Mum's, which the real estate agent had begun to showcase as 'the homeliest room in the village'.

I wonder how they picked each other out. Their studios were close by and they'd meet up in the lounge and dining room as long as Mum ventured out. But they couldn't consciously build a friendship in the usual ways: sharing confidences, pursuing common interests, making plans. Yet somehow they recognised a kindred spirit in each other and became almost inseparable.

The first time I met Lesla, she told me how nice my hair looked. I said I'd just made an appointment to get it cut.

'Cancel it!' she ordered, slicing the air with her hand. The next time I saw her, she told me again how nice my hair looked. Mischievously, I gave the same answer to see how she'd respond.

'Cancel it!' she said with the same fruity laugh.

It became a ritual, reassuring in its predictability: her compliment, my hair appointment, her command to cancel it. I wondered if she really liked my hair or whether, like Mum (like all of us), she had a stock of social niceties that passed for conversation.

Lesla's upbeat nature brought out the best in Mum. In the lull between Christmas and New Year, I took the pair of them to see *Out of the Blue* at The Embassy, the renamed cinema where I'd lost the chic blue shoulder bag on my eleventh birthday. The movie was about New Zealand's worst-ever shooting spree, in Aramoana, a small coastal settlement near Dunedin. (It seems an odd choice, I agree.) Afterwards, we went upstairs to the café for coffee and cake.

'Well, that was a very powerful film,' Lesla said, emptying her handbag onto the table for the third time to check she had her wallet.

Mum nodded. 'It's a long time since I got a hanky out at the movies. Pip's the one who always cries.' Perhaps triggered by this thought, or by the South Island setting of the movie, she began to reminisce about the horrors of being a boarder again. Crying herself to sleep at night. The 'unbelievable' strictness. Always being watched.

Every Saturday at six o'clock was 'Rules': when the nuns read out the week's infringements and punishments.

'Punishments for what?' I asked.

'Ridiculous things. Talking. Going outside without a note. Not eating your dinner.'

Once again I was struck by the resemblance to the retirement village. When Mum tried to walk outside, she'd told me, a staff member called, 'Mrs Desmond, Mrs Desmond, where do you think you're going?' It wasn't as if she could wander far: she was much too unsteady. Not like Lorna who'd recently been found four kilometres away on the Ngauranga Gorge exit road, heading towards six lanes of traffic.

Many of Mum's angry notes related to eating: the 'Hundred Years' War', to borrow Atul Gawande's phrase, where the battle for control between institution and resident plays out. 'I couldn't eat a disgusting Bread and Butter pudding tonight (took me back to boarding school days so left it) so R and/or supervisor will be complaining to you about me (just warning you),' said one, referring specifically to those dreadful desserts at St Dom's.

'I don't want to talk about it, it still upsets me,' she said about the punishments. She paused. 'Oh, I suppose it didn't do me any harm.'

'Those memories go pretty deep, don't they?' I said, trying to keep them flowing.

She gave me an anxious look. 'It didn't make me hard on you, did it?'

'No, Mum.' *Not till you got dementia.*

'Well, that was a very powerful film,' Lesla said.

Mum nodded. 'It's a long time since I got a hanky out at the movies. Pip's the one who always cries.'

CHAPTER EIGHTEEN

HOME VISIT

'COMPARED TO OCTOBER, it feels like my sisters all have so much more "new" time that used to be spent worrying about whether Mum was OK, who was checking up on her, and whether they should try and fit in another rushed, stressful visit to Colville St,' Matt emailed while he was home in January 2007. For all the retirement village's shortcomings, it had freed us from the quicksand of Mum's household affairs. It had also changed the pecking order. Now it was Kate who lived near Mum and could pop in at short notice. Her nursing background gave her the confidence to shower Mum when she rebuffed the staff, to check on her medication, talk to the manager. Kate's four-year-old daughter Sarah adored Mum, a feeling that was reciprocal.

In the same email, Matt suggested putting Colville Street on the market. His reasons were sound: it was better to sell over summer; the house would need a refit if we left it much longer; if we didn't sell, we'd have to go through the hassle of finding paying tenants.

'This will probably be shattering news for Mum,' he

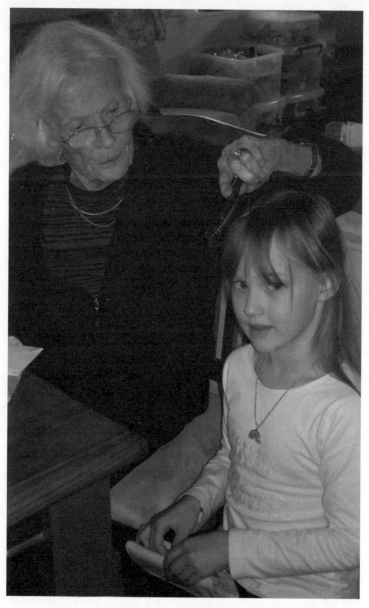

Mum with her youngest grandchild Sarah, 2008.
They shared a mutual devotion.

acknowledged. 'If we do go ahead, we will need lots of mutual support and a united front. I can play the "bad cop" if we can make a decision in the next week or so . . . I think that we need to get very clear again on where we are all going with this. That Mum will find it easier to move on if we stop the "therapeutic fibbing" and ensure there are as few mixed messages as possible. She is easily sharp enough (and desperate enough) to exploit them.'

None of us seriously believed that Mum would live at Colville Street again. But it was a huge step to dispose of the house she hadn't seen since we'd bundled her off to hospital. Nor would Matt be around to pack up 50 years of accumulated possessions or oversee the process.

'We can simplify it as much as possible but there will still be a lot involved — trust me,' replied Rose, who was in the throes of selling her own house. I had my own reason for not wanting to rush things. Avah was barely three months old. I knew Megan and Rome couldn't stay there forever but I wanted to give them a bit longer.

This time it was my big brother who put up with my tears and helped me navigate my fractured loyalties to my daughter, my mother and my siblings. I decided to opt out of the family meeting to discuss the sale, and the others accepted Matt's time frame.

That night I dreamed I arrived at Colville Street to find an 'open home' sign outside and a crowd of people partying on the back deck. I scurried past, hoping no one would see me. Then I was drinking tea with Mum in the retirement village lounge. She set off down the stairs to the dining room. I tried to follow her but got waylaid by another resident. When I turned back, Mum was heading out a side door. I hurried after her into a crowded outdoor market. As she walked briskly between ramshackle stalls, too far ahead for me to call out, it dawned on me that she had no idea where she was going. She had got us both lost.

IN SPITE OF Liz's efforts to head Mum off by ringing her at breakfast every morning, my Saturday began with four angry phone calls. I imagined Mum sitting at her table in her blue silk dressing gown, gazing out at the hills and harbour, thumbing through the morning paper while she sipped the tea she complained was always cold. Then triggered by something — what? — picking up her phone and dialling my number to accuse me of incarcerating her. Over and over again. Until I stopped taking her calls and left her to berate the answer machine.

I bolted my muesli and went to get her. When I told her it was chilly outside, she put on a second blouse over the one she was wearing. Combing her wispy hair in the mirror, she noticed the blouse and took it off again. Then she aimed a can of hairspray at her hair. A thin film settled on her glasses. I tried to wash it off with soap and made a mental note to tackle it with something stronger when we got home; her balance was bad enough without her being blind too.

As we drove past Wellington Hospital where her fate had been sealed, Mum asked me to take her to Colville Street. I said it wasn't a good time; that Megan's children were asleep.

'I'll be very quiet,' she said, breaking my heart all over again.

'Let's go to the bottle store first,' I said, invoking the therapeutic fibbing principle of distraction. By the time we'd replenished the gin and wine that her friends demolished at speed, she'd forgotten her request.

At home we sat in the sun and let Pat cheer us up. But as soon as he went inside, Mum started on me again.

'I've seen your name on the form at reception,' she said. 'You've signed me in for eight weeks.'

'Where would you like to live?' I asked.

'Now you're being tricky,' she said, which of course was true.

'Remember how hard it was looking after Dad at home?' I said, hoping to tap into her empathy.

'Yes,' she said coldly. 'And I didn't carry on like this. And I looked after my mother.' She glared at me. 'You just want to get rid of the problem. Rose is very sorry about the predicament I find myself in.'

Pitting me against my little sister undermined all my good intentions. I told Mum she had to lay off me, it wasn't my fault. Then I asked Pat to drive her back to the village — I couldn't face one more car ride with her.

After a sleepless night, I emailed my siblings to say I wanted to take Mum back to Colville Street. If she was angry afterwards, it didn't matter: she was angry now. I sympathised with her: she'd had to leave her home abruptly and had never been back. I said it would be good if one of them came too, and it was all right if they thought I was the wrong person as long as someone else did it. I also said I'd be willing to take her back as many times as she wanted until the house was sold.

Kate offered to come with me. On a grey afternoon in late March, five months after Mum had left her house, she walked back in as if she'd just popped down to the supermarket. Megan and Rome had taken the children out, leaving the house so shipshape Mum thought they'd gone for good. She was proprietorial, comfortable, delighted. It still felt like her house — it even smelled like hers. She could move back in 'on Wednesday', she suggested.

Stiff-legged and hunched in her brown fleecy jacket, Mum scuttled from room to room like a sandpiper. Of all her knick-knacks, it was the artificial red carnations in a green glass vase and the pots on the back deck that caught her eye. There wasn't much left in the way of colour except a fuchsia with fat pink and purple flowers. But Megan, who'd inherited her grandmother's green fingers, had pruned and staked things and transplanted the green and silver flax from around the front into a terracotta pot. 'It looks so much better, not so cramped,' Mum said approvingly.

We sat in the lounge. Immediately, Mum wanted to light the fire and turn the heaters on full, reminding me of those $100-a-week power bills. Kate shared an easy patter with Mum that I seemed to have lost. She asked her about the Roxburgh souvenirs dotted around the room. Several — a black water buffalo, an embroidered bird print, the green pottery jar Mum had kept buttons in after the pickled ginger was gone — were gifts from Henry Ah Chee, Mum said. He'd been a school friend of her father's and later the Chinese consul to New Zealand. In return, John Harry would send Henry a box of cherries from the Waigth & Sons orchard every Christmas.

Recalling her childhood, Mum's voice grew stronger and her eyes brightened, as if drawing energy from the past made her feel more alive in the present. She'd always been proud of the two men's friendship — and of John Harry's relationship with the generally maligned Chinese labourers on his orchard. I knew the strait-laced National Party stalwart had gone so far as to buy them opium from Kempthorne Prosser in Dunedin under the guise of orchard supplies. Mum told me he'd shown Dad the record in his business ledger.

She remembered an opium pipe stored on a high shelf in the family wash house too. When I asked if her father might have used it, she'd laughed. 'A memento probably.' In the Waigth household, tobacco was a no-no, drinking meant a sherry after dinner.

Hong, one of the orchard labourers, became the family gardener. In Mum's albums, there's a photo of him sitting on the back lawn in work boots and a brimmed hat. Beside him perches Mum, a toddler, on a wooden plank. They're both holding cups: it must be smoko. They couldn't be more different, the little girl in the white dress and ankle socks, and the dark-skinned man so far from home. Yet they seem comfortable with each other and stare at the camera with the same solemn intensity.

Not much else sparked Mum's interest: a cluster of side tables from her mother, some second-hand items she'd bought when she and Dad moved to Wellington, the standing lamp with the curved, flowered base 'which was very expensive'.

In the study we sat again. Mum ignored Dad's desk, the former site of her paper panic, and expressed alarm at the stack of books on the floor from the bookcase we'd taken to her studio. What would she do with them if the house was sold, she asked?

We reassured her that we'd pack them up and suggested she go downstairs, holding back to see how she'd manage. She teetered at the top, then grabbed the bannister and sailed down as easily as she always had. In her bedroom, Kate helped Mum choose some winter outfits from among the skirts, blouses and trousers that hung in a wardrobe as orderly as a fashion store. Mum's good habits had helped us keep her at Colville Street; I feared for my family if it came down to a question of mine.

Her clothes were generally pastels, beige, olive green, sometimes navy blue. 'You're too young to wear black,' she'd tell me, a rule she still applied to herself. A long time ago, she'd worked out what suited her — muted colours, clean lines, timeless styles — and stuck to it. Which was why she always looked so good.

Mum whipped things on and off with an agility as surprising as her lack of inhibition. Some of the garments had mildew from months of sitting in the cold room, and they all smelled musty, reminding me why we needed to sell the house. I spied a pair of black knickers underneath her white ones, and a tissue tucked into the elastic. Her thighs were the same width as her knees; her ankles fatter than both.

From time to time she announced she was moving out of the retirement village. But when we suggested she look for a bigger apartment — our new tactic — she told us there weren't any and her studio was very sunny and the village was quite good and the worst thing was the way it had been done behind her back. She even wrote Megan a note saying how beautifully she'd looked after Colville Street and praising her baby photos. I hoped it would make up for the awful phone calls my daughter had to field.

Throughout the afternoon I took photos so Mum would remember she'd been there. As we were leaving, I suggested she stand at the front door for a final shot. She clasped her hands behind her back and wouldn't look at me. She looked so lonely that I told Kate to go and stand with her.

When Mum turned to the camera, her eyes were accusing, her mouth set in a straight line. Then her face crumpled. 'If I look at the photo later, I'll cry,' she said through strangled sobs. I rushed up to her and put my arms around her. She buried her head in my chest, then pulled back. I took her inside and sat her in the lounge again.

'I'm sorry,' she kept saying, angry with herself for breaking down.

'You don't have to apologise,' I said. 'It's really sad. You're allowed to cry.'

'No. If I start, I'll never stop.' But the sobs kept coming anyway.

I crouched in front of her and stroked her knee. Then Kate was behind me jollying us both along. Somehow Mum got back to the story about the five men in the dining room whose wives were glad to be rid of them and I wondered whose side she was on now.

Later I wished I'd responded with some 'Sorrys' of my own. *Sorry I can't make you better, Mum. Sorry I can't take you home. Sorry I can't look after you like you looked after Dad and Grandma. Sorry my love is not enough. Sorry, sorry, sorry.* I put some of this in an email to my siblings.

'Mum is and always has been a pragmatist,' Kate replied. 'Yes, she was sad at Colville St, but there's a part of her that knows it's for the best. Remember the way she left Wadestown Rd? And she has some good times at the village. She came for tea last night and regaled everyone with the good things about it — including the soirées in each other's rooms — and how she's selling Colville St — totally matter of fact.'

Ah, the different mothers again. And the different daughters.

CHAPTER NINETEEN

———

A PRAYER

AUSTRALIAN DEMENTIA ACTIVIST Christine Bryden gave a public talk. I'm not sure why I went to hear her; I generally didn't want to know what lay ahead for Mum. If I'd known Christine had early onset Alzheimer's disease, I'd have been even less inclined: dementia felt particularly confronting when it claimed people younger than myself.

Christine was a pale, attractive woman in her mid-fifties who'd been a biochemist. She seemed warm and serene, although she compared herself to a duck paddling flat out under the surface to appear normal.

Her quality of life depended on three things, she said: her Christian faith, the love of her husband Paul and her daughters, and drugs, particularly the drug Aricept. Its benefits were so profound she had an agreement with Paul to give it to her till she died, she said — a reminder that the time would come when she wouldn't be able to enforce that choice herself.

Mum had been taking Aricept for nearly a year and we often

wondered if it was doing any good. We were in the trap that Carol from Alzheimers Wellington had warned us about. It wasn't until you took the expensive drug away that you found out if it had been helping, she said. She'd seen families devastated when a parent went downhill quickly, maybe losing the ability to speak — and there was no going back.

When Christine called for questions, I asked her if she recommended Aricept for people with vascular dementia, for whom there was less evidence it helped than for Alzheimer's disease.

She thought for a moment. 'People I know take it,' she said, then moved on to the next question. As I was considering this deceptively simple statement, a group of elderly people shuffled in through a side door. To my horror, Mum was among them. I realised she must be on an outing with the Marsden Club, the Chelsea Club's sister service on her new side of town. I sank down in my chair, feeling like a secret agent whose cover's been blown. I hoped she hadn't heard my question.

When the session was over, I took Mum a cup of tea, afraid that she'd ask me what I was doing there — or what she was. But she was more concerned about the club member sitting lopsided in the next seat, chin lolling on her chest, noisily sucking in air. 'She's a bit grim,' Mum said out of the corner of her mouth.

Across the room I caught sight of an acquaintance, Kate, a vibrant woman in her late forties. I waved and she made her way through the crowd. 'I've got early Alzheimer's too,' she said.

I knew that. When the disease had forced her to give up her job a few years earlier, my minister at Parliament had asked me to find her some work in our office. I'd sat with Kate in front of a computer to get her started on some data entry.

'Click on the file name,' I'd said.

'How do I do that?' she asked.

'Just push your index finger down on the mouse.' I showed her. She pushed her finger down.

'Now click at the top of the first column.'

'How do I do that?' she asked again.

I showed her. She pushed her finger down.

'Now click at the top of the next column.'

'How do I do that?'

This was my first experience of dementia close up and it took me a while to realise that Kate would never remember how to open a file, no matter how many times I showed her. That day she'd seemed brittle and nervous. Now she was tanned and confident, although her blue eyes had lost most of their sparkle. She'd spent the first year after her diagnosis being really sad, she said, and the second being really angry. Then she stopped fighting the disease, learned to move towards it rather than backing away. Mixing with others who had Alzheimer's helped. Like Christine, she was putting her people skills to good use as a spokesperson for the disease.

It took me a long time to realise that the difference between these two women and Mum, apart from their age, was their insight. They knew what was wrong with them, were involved in decisions about their illness and had a community of support. That's why Christine's statement, 'People I know take it', was so profound, I realised. Those people had vascular dementia, they'd decided Aricept was worth taking and they'd talked it over with Christine.

Mum, on the other hand, had no idea what was wrong with her, except for occasional flashes. She wasn't in denial. She wasn't being wilful or obtuse. Hard as it is to comprehend, many — maybe most — people with dementia don't know they've got it. They can't remember that they can't remember. It's a feature of the disease. It even has a name: anosognosia.

On the surface, it may seem like a blessing to be spared the horror of knowing you're losing your mind. But in my experience, it's the hardest thing about dementia. It makes the job of caregivers heartbreakingly difficult and conflict-ridden. And it locks sufferers into a private hell, believing the world and those they love have turned against them.

Describing pain in general in an online meditation summit in 2016, American Buddhist nun Pema Chodron notes that 'the sense of isolation gets so strong, the sense of our particular, personal burden and the loneliness of that and the desperation of that.' Healing is to be found in community and kinship, she says. 'There's something enormously comforting about being able to say, "Other people feel this". That sounds so simplistic but, believe me, it makes a big difference.'

Mum didn't know other people felt like her. She couldn't even name her illness, let alone make sense of it. In the absence of wider support, she clung to us, her children. Our task — perhaps our most important task — was to reassure her she was not alone.

MUM PHONED ME three times in a row, each time more agitated. Vague claims that she'd been dumped and abandoned gave way to tears that she'd had to eat lunch by herself in the dining room. This seemed doubtful but I rang the charge nurse to ask her to check on Mum. It was only when I asked if anything had happened to upset her that the nurse admitted there'd been 'a small problem' at lunch. Too many of the women wanted to sit together. She'd had to ask Mum to move out of someone else's chair.

I'd witnessed the nurse's brusque manner and knew how humiliated Mum would have felt at being singled out in public. Putting aside the issue of why Mum didn't have her own chair, I asked who she'd sat with after that.

The nurse named a married couple.

Did Mum know them, I asked? As far as I could tell, she and Lesla were part of a small group, all women, who trotted around like a flock of sheep and were easily startled and scattered.

'She should,' said the nurse. 'They live on the same floor as her.' She sounded defensive. 'We had to do something. It was only a minor issue.'

'Not in Mum's mind,' I said. I asked her not to tell Mum I'd phoned: she might think I'd got her into trouble. For all I knew, I had. The nurse was just as likely to scold her as calm her down. It reminded me of going in to bat for my kids at school, never knowing if I'd make things worse. But at least my kids got to come home at night and could tell me what had happened during the day.

I also asked the nurse to get Lesla to look in on Mum. If anyone could cheer her up, it was her optimistic friend. I have no idea if she did. She never let me know and I felt too intimidated to ask. By the time I phoned Mum back, she'd forgotten about the lunch incident but it showed up for days in her unsettled behaviour. As Rose observed, 'When Mum doesn't feel she belongs at the village, she just wants to go home.'

A PIECE OF paper fell out of Mum's diary. On it she'd written the prayer that begins, 'Every day I need you, Lord, but this day especially, I need some extra strength to face whatever is to be.' I wondered whether something new had happened to upset her or if she'd had a glimpse of the future. Generally she had little time for religious platitudes.

A resident approached us as Mum signed herself out at reception. 'Does anyone know what day it is?' she asked in a plummy voice.

I told her it was Sunday.

'Damn, I haven't been to Mass,' she said.

'Don't worry,' Mum chipped in. 'God will understand.' She'd always been a devout Catholic. But these days her God was less of a stickler for the rules, or perhaps less relevant altogether.

'It's not just about God,' the woman said. 'I've been to Mass every Sunday for my whole life.'

'It's all right, Val, you can go next week,' Mum said.

'My name's not Val.'

Mum's brow wrinkled. 'Mary?'

'I answer to most things but actually it's Kay.'

'There are so many new people in here, it's impossible to keep up,' Mum said airily.

She was becoming an old hand. 'Every day I found Mum (totally forgetful of our plans) cosily involved in some activity or other,' Liz emailed after a trip to Wellington in April, six months after Mum moved into the village. 'Once I had the chance to sit at the back and watch while she played indoor bowls and she seemed really relaxed and happy.' (The activities officer told us she had such a good eye and arm that her nickname was 'Smash'.) 'When I found her squished up on the couch with three others, chatting away about nothing, on Tuesday, I couldn't help but think of all the lonely hours at Colville St,' Liz added.

We'd taken Mum back several times by then. Liz also took her to see the lawyer, a formality to legitimise the sale of the house in her mind since Rose and I had joint power of attorney. When the lawyer asked her about the retirement village, 'Mum had nothing but praise', Liz said. 'She said that she's been there for 8 years now! The magical figure 8, eh!'

I don't know why Mum chose to measure her new life in increments of eight unless there was some connection to our family of eight. But it was heartening to see her stronger and happier. 'Had a lovely day today with Mum,' Ginny emailed. 'A little girl was dancing merrily on the lawn at the Botanical Gardens which reminded Mum of us doing the same. Off to church and she caught up with lots of parishioners and on to dinner at One Red Dog on the wharf — fantastic weather. All that fresh air. I'm sure she'll sleep well.'

Lesla can take much of the credit for Mum's new contentment.

'She's been the saving grace of this place,' Mum confided. 'I don't think I'd have survived without her.' Ditto.

When we took Mum out, we'd often scoop up her best friend as well. 'The conversation in the car went around and around on the same subjects, quite funny and neither of them noticed any repetition,' Ginny emailed after a trip to the wind turbine. On the way back, they stopped to watch Ginny's teenage Asian sons play tennis against two middle-aged European men. 'Lesla says to me, "Now, which two are yours?" T'was hard to keep a straight face.'

As for the prayer about needing extra strength, my sisters were less moved than me. Kate: 'Yep, it's been in Mum's diary a week or so. I left that and removed another rave about Colville St (!) Both written in the most beautiful, neat, legible handwriting that I've seen in a long time.'

And Rose: 'I don't really remember Mum being quite into that stuff but she is surrounded by Catholics!!'

CHAPTER TWENTY

ACTS OF KINDNESS

LESLA LOOKED UP from her newspaper when I put my head around her studio door.

'You haven't got Mum in there, have you?' I asked. I'd brought my friend Annie to see her — she'd known Mum since we were in our twenties.

'Not unless she's hiding under the bed.' Lesla smiled. 'Your hair's looking very nice today.'

'Damn, I've just made an appointment to get it cut.'

'Cancel it!'

We both laughed.

Mum was nowhere to be found. It was Sunday and the carers' station was vacant. I checked the day book and saw Mum had signed herself out but there was nothing to say where she'd gone or with whom. Finally a resident told me she'd left with a man and another woman. I wondered if they'd let anyone kidnap these forgetful old birds.

Annie and I drove to Makara. As we walked around the rocky coast, we talked about the book I was still writing long after my university course had finished. It was Annie who'd introduced me to the Wellington gang scene in the 1970s and persuaded me to help her set up Aroha Trust, a work cooperative for young women. We'd been through a lot together and she couldn't turn me down when I asked to record her story for the book, along with those of 11 other women. I'd promised I wouldn't use anything they told me without their permission. Still, she was anxious about public exposure of their lives.

'When are you going to show us all a draft?' she asked.

'Labour Weekend, I hope.'

'I'll be there,' she said.

'You'd better be.'

On our way back we called into the village again and found Mum sitting in the lounge. She looked smart in striped cotton trousers and the high-necked top she only changed under duress. She smiled and waved when she saw us. My stomach unclenched to see her in a good mood. I made sure I said Annie's name in case she'd forgotten it.

'How lovely to see you, Annie,' Mum said. 'How long has it been?' What a clever question, I thought, if you were trying to work out where someone fitted in your life.

'Six or seven years,' Annie said. 'Me and some of the other Aroha Trust women came to your house. We were starving and we ate all your cheese and crackers.'

'The things you remember,' Mum said. She turned to the woman sitting beside her. 'This is—'

'Clare,' the woman said.

'I hear you two have been out for lunch with a man,' I said.

Mum looked at Clare. 'Where did we go? Isn't that awful? It was only a few hours ago.'

'Waikanae?' Clare suggested.

Mum nodded. 'In the bus.'

A staff member walked past. 'Tea in ten minutes,' she said.

'We've got our marching orders,' said Clare in a low voice.

'You don't have to go yet,' I said.

'No,' said Mum. 'We just end up waiting around down there.' She began asking Annie what she'd been doing with herself and Annie told her, unaware that her answers were as ephemeral for Mum as a puff of smoke.

The door from the studio corridor swung open and Lorna appeared, wringing her hands. As soon as she reached us, she turned around. 'I have to go back, I've left the fire burning in my room,' she said.

I watched, helpless, as she rushed away to deal with the imaginary flames.

Clare stood up. 'She's had an upset, I need to look after her,' she said.

Mum seemed unfazed by the kerfuffle. 'Catherine rang me the other night,' she said. Catherine was Lorna's daughter. 'Lorna has a very bad memory problem. She's meant to be having brain surgery, but she's refusing. I can't say I blame her.'

'Me neither,' I said.

Out of nowhere, Mum's face clouded over. 'Catherine said *you* told her I was in here and that's why they decided to put Lorna here too.'

In fact, it had been the other way round. 'Maybe Catherine saw you when she visited Lorna one day,' I suggested.

'No, *you* told her.' Mum's voice was hard; she seemed to be blaming me for Lorna's downfall as well as her own.

I couldn't help myself. 'But Lorna moved in months before you,' I protested.

'Well then, Catherine must have moved very fast,' Mum said, reversing time without apology.

We walked Mum to the lift where a crowd milled around the

door. As it opened, an elderly man took her arm with a 'C'mon, Rosaleen!' while the woman with him turned to me and said, 'Don't worry, we'll look after her. She sits at our table.' This must be the married couple Mum had been made to eat lunch with in the dining room. They seemed solicitous and charming, a reminder that while Mum couldn't tell us when she'd been bullied, she couldn't remember acts of kindness either.

Annie didn't seem to have noticed Mum's sudden funk. 'Your mother's better than I expected,' she said on the way out. 'Isn't it nice she went on the bus with her friend to Waikanae today?'

I stopped in the middle of the foyer. 'Annie, we have no idea where they went. Or who with. Or how they got there. It certainly wasn't on the bus. There is no bus trip on Sundays.'

'Are you sure?'

'I'm positive.'

Annie fell about laughing. 'Well, they had me fooled.'

I managed a grin. 'Welcome to my world.'

The following weekend, I ran into an old family friend, Bernard, on the sideline of Jackson's rugby game. He asked if Mum had enjoyed her Sunday outing. Another mystery benefactor revealed.

ON A WINTRY night in July, Mum phoned to say she'd been told to be in her pyjamas and in bed by eight-thirty because the doctor was coming to put cream in her eye. There was nothing wrong with her eye, she said. She didn't want to go to bed early.

I understood her reluctance. It was bad enough that residents were served dinner at five o'clock every night like small children, at odds with the rhythms of the adult world. Evenings yawned ahead of them without organised activities and almost no staff on duty. These oldies didn't need much sleep but couldn't concentrate on TV, reading or hobbies. What got them through the long, empty hours was each other. Now Mum felt she'd been banished to her studio to face the night alone.

I asked her to put the carer on the phone. A heavily accented voice told me Mum's eye had been red and itchy that morning. The doctor had just faxed through a prescription. It was best if Mum got ready for bed because the ointment was sticky and she might not be able to see properly afterwards.

'But it's not sore now,' Mum said, taking the phone back. 'And I've never seen the doctor.' This may have been true, I decided: surely he wouldn't have faxed through the prescription if he'd been on site. She wanted a second opinion. 'Wouldn't you, Pip?'

Before I could reply, I heard a muffled exchange, then a door bang. Mum came back on the line. 'I can't stand that woman, she always shouts at me,' she said, a little breathless and excited.

I realised she'd shut the carer out of the studio. I told her I needed to check with Kate, who confirmed the sore eye. We agreed the staff should abandon the ointment overnight.

Mum sounded grateful and rather smug when I rang her back. Feeling like a mediator in a hostage situation, I asked to speak to the carer again.

The woman seemed shaken. 'I didn't want to do the ointment in front of everyone but your Mum stormed back into the group and said I was making her go to bed early. You'd think I'd be used to it after three and a half years.' She sounded close to tears. The new carer she'd been training had also been upset by Mum's shouting, she said.

I apologised, wondering where her supervisor was and why I was having to manage this stand-off over the phone.

'We still have to get your mother's sleeping pill into her,' the carer said. 'I think I'll ask someone else to do it.'

'Don't worry, Mum loves her sleeping pill,' I said.

'I'll still ask someone else.'

I found myself feeling sorry for the woman. I'd often thought it would be easier to deal with dementia without the emotional baggage attached to being a daughter. Now I realised the baggage buoyed me up as much as it weighed me down. I had suitcases full of memories, love, gratitude and family ties to draw on. The carers at the retirement village were paid low wages to be overworked, unsupported and shouted at by strangers. Almost all were immigrant women, looking after their adopted society's old people, one of the few jobs they could get. It said a lot about the value we accorded both groups. One or two managed to win Mum over with natural skill and empathy, but most had no idea how to handle her. They lacked communication skills and cultural understanding, in-depth training, strategies, back-up. The words 'real estate, not health care' rang in my ears.

When I saw Mum two days later, her eyes were better — without the ointment. Which just left all the other medication she was on. Kate found a day's supply of pills sitting on Mum's dresser: Aricept for dementia, Felodipine for blood pressure, Omeprazole for nausea, Fosamax for bone density, Triazolam for sleeping, plus a multivitamin. The charge nurse assured Kate the oversight was rare. Mum hated being watched while she took her pills, which was staff policy, and the nurse hadn't wanted to be too forceful, she said — although that didn't explain why the pills had been left behind for Mum to do whatever she liked with them.

A week later Rose found an even greater stockpile. When she pointed the pills out to Mum, Mum wanted to take the lot then and there.

'My first reaction is to make a written complaint but I suppose we have to tread carefully knowing how that could backfire on Mum and also knowing how obstreperous Mum can be,' Liz emailed. 'I mean, what should the carers do if she refuses to take them? It needs a whole-team approach which the village is sadly lacking.'

We requested a meeting with the nursing manager. She agreed to send a carer back later if Mum refused to take her pills, and to monitor the situation weekly. It was depressing to think this wasn't already the case.

CHAPTER TWENTY-ONE

ALIVE INSIDE

AFTER A FLURRY of real estate agent visits, working bees and repairs, gardening and tree-topping, open homes and weekends spent emptying Colville Street's 12 rooms, in August 2007 we gratefully accepted the only offer to buy the house. By then we'd taken Mum back a number of times but she showed little interest in its contents or demise.

Lesla's accident the same month had a bigger impact. 'Mum is absolutely certain she saw Lesla fall over that lady's legs, when and how,' Rose emailed. 'What a memory!'

Lesla broke her hip and was transferred to a public hospital. Rose took Mum to visit her. 'We had a lovely old time and Mum seemed pretty with it, if a little subdued,' she said. 'The circular conversation centring on the view from the window didn't bother either of them. Mum kept reiterating how much everyone was missing Lesla and they all send their love, to which Lesla must have replied at least 6 times: "Well, just send it right back. Oh, that sounds a bit rude!!"'

When she came back to the village, Lesla went into the hospital wing to recuperate. Occasionally we'd take Mum to see her, but Mum couldn't find her way to the hospital alone and the gulf between their lives widened. Soon afterwards Lorna was transferred to the rest home and Mum lost another mooring. Within six months, both her friends — who'd seemed so much more robust than her — had died.

In uncertain times, Mum's anger ramped up. She kept telling me I'd incarcerated her, an accusation I found impossible to strip of its emotional sting. I tried to invoke the therapeutic fibbing model: reassure, don't argue, tell compassionate lies. I did this with my heart in my mouth. Anxious Mum would catch me out. Bereft when she didn't.

One day I decided that the next time she said she might as well be dead, I'd offer to take her home to live with me. This would reassure her that I loved her, that I understood her fear and loneliness; she wouldn't remember when I didn't keep my word. But I could never bring myself to say it. Some things are too big to lie about. If I made such a promise and broke it, I believed Mum would feel even more abandoned, if only at an unconscious level.

I wish I knew if that were true.

TO OUR RELIEF and admiration, Mum made another new friend. Marie didn't lift Mum's spirits in the way Lesla had: we'd often find the pair of them huddled on the couch like refugees, bemoaning their fate. Still, having a buddy boosted Mum's confidence and well-being.

As she approached her seventy-eighth birthday and one-year

anniversary at the village, the GP pronounced her in perfect health. 'Mum was positively beaming,' Ginny emailed. He assured her a growth on her hand wouldn't cause any problems for five to 10 years. 'By which time I'll be dead,' Mum replied.

The same day, Mum heated a wheat bag in the microwave without a glass of water for so long that it exploded and hurled scorched kernels all over her room. But her pitiful weight was more or less stable, her nausea and back pain more or less manageable; her mood more or less benign. In the seven months between September 2007 and April 2008, our email barometer dropped to 18, an all-time low; there were only five in the month before Christmas, so fraught the previous year.

On Saturday mornings over the summer I began taking advantage of Mum's half-price taxi fares to save me the hour round-trip to pick her up. Masterminding the operation often took just as long, but at least I could make muffins at the same time. First I'd ring Mum to tell her to put on her jacket and start making her way to the front entrance. Then I'd ring the cab company, describe Mum, tell them she had dementia and ask them to get the driver to contact me if there was a problem.

Things got tricky once Mum left her studio. From the other side of town I'd will her to walk down the corridor, through the lounge, into the foyer and out the front door without getting waylaid. During this time she was as unreachable as if she were trekking in the Tararua Ranges. There was no one to escort her. On Saturdays, the skeleton staff was so stretched showering and dressing residents that they rarely answered the phone. Once I got through to a carer and she agreed to put Mum in a cab, then forgot. In Mum's notes the carer says, 'Mrs Desmond's daughter was very angry.'

One morning in the New Year, the cab driver rang to say Mum wasn't waiting outside as arranged. I called her studio landline but there was no answer. I asked him to go inside and look for her, wondering how he'd pick her out from all the other small,

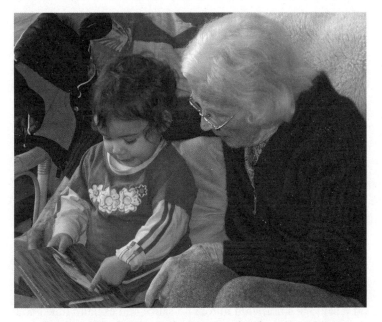

One-year-old Avah entertains her great-grandmother, 2008. 'Megan, you have such beautiful children,' Mum would say over and over again.

wandering, white-haired women. Fifteen minutes later, he let me know they were on their way.

Outside our gate, the driver opened the cab door for Mum and she stepped out, waving like royalty. As I handed over a small fortune for his 45-minute search and rescue mission, he said, 'Enjoy your birthday celebration, your mother's really looking forward to it.'

'I will,' said I whose birthday is in August.

Those Saturday mornings are some of my happiest memories of this time: four generations gathered in our backyard, tui swooping in to feast on the kōwhai, the pine forest a wavy green ocean along the skyline. Mum's grandchildren would fuss over her and make her laugh. Her great-grandchildren cared nothing about muddled brains or brittle bones.

'Megan, you have such beautiful children,' Mum would say as they snuggled up beside her in shorts and sunhats while she read them *The Hungry Caterpillar* and *Goodnight, Moon.* Long after they'd toddled off to pick fresh peas from the garden and ferret for strawberries, she'd stare at the picture books, oblivious to their squeals as my boys swung them upside down.

Sometimes Pat would fire up Barbie, our new brick barbecue that had all but replaced me in his affections. Mum would polish off a sausage smothered in tomato sauce and exclaim how good food tasted when it was cooked outdoors. 'Someone else's bread and butter,' she'd say, her stock compliment for a meal, however humble, that she hadn't had to prepare herself.

But then the entertainment would go home and Mum would start fretting that she needed to get back to the village she hated. One afternoon, I took her for a drive to distract her. Wellington was doing its four-seasons-in-a-day thing and, by the time we got to Seatoun, a pesky breeze wrecked any chance of getting her out of the car. In the front seat we licked Trumpets and watched kids dive off the rickety wharf, their legs splayed like frogs. A young man with a windsurfer pulled himself up, hauled his sail out of the waves, and fell off, time and time again. I wanted to be out there too, feeling the spray on my face, learning new tricks, not cooped up in a car like a 78-year-old.

I waited until I was driving Mum back to her studio to bring up a difficult subject. Teenagers had taught me the car's an ideal place for awkward conversations: no eye contact; no means of escape; no room for histrionics. Rose's friend's mother — the one at her fiftieth birthday party who had vascular dementia and had gone to live with her son — had recently contracted pneumonia. She recovered after being given antibiotics but the illness took a toll and she was now in a dementia unit. We needed to know what Mum thought about medical intervention if she got sick.

I told her this story and suggested it could be hard sometimes to decide whether to use antibiotics.

'What do you mean?' she said sharply.

I reminded her that Dad, or perhaps she on his behalf, had refused antibiotics for pneumonia when he was terminally ill.

'Well, he'd been sick for a—' She paused. 'Very. Long. Time.' She stressed the last three words to remind me that she hadn't. I had my answer. Life force, survival instinct, lack of insight. Whatever the reason, Mum had no intention of opting out early, regardless of how unhappy she claimed to be, or how much we might want to protect her from a fate we feared might be worse than death.

'He just got worn out,' she said after a silence. 'When he got sick, he still had so much left to do. It wasn't fair. I used to look up there sometimes' — she tilted her eyes towards the roof — 'and say, "*What* do you think you're doing?"' It was the most eloquent I'd heard her for a long time — and the most poignant. She might accept God's grand design but she was not above challenging his poorer calls.

As Liz pointed out, though, it wouldn't be Mum who made the decision about medical intervention; it would be us. We scurried away to give more thought to the ethics. I used to believe human beings weren't wise enough to choose their own moment of death. Now I'm not sure that nature, boosted by science, is either.

Mum only had dementia for a fraction of the time that Dad was sick. But the experience of caring for her shook my Catholic-based certainty in the sanctity of life in a way that his brain tumour hadn't. That's partly because I wasn't his main caregiver and partly because the tumour didn't fundamentally change who he was.

I can't see the compassion — or point — in keeping someone alive if their essence is gone. The difficulty, of course, is knowing when that has happened. There's a YouTube clip about the power of music to rouse even those with advanced dementia, part of a documentary called *Alive Inside*. Henry, 94, sits in his wheelchair, slumped and unresponsive. That's how he used to spend his days until a perceptive social worker gave him headphones and played his favourite Cab Calloway songs through them.

We see the headphones go on, Henry's face light up, his eyes bug out. His body moves and he starts to sing; he still knows all the words. 'It gives me the feeling of love,' he says when asked what the music does. Henry's in there after all — and apparently he came out for Cab Calloway right up until his death.

An aunt on Dad's side who had Alzheimer's disease could hit the high notes of 'Ave Maria' long after she couldn't string a sentence together; Glen Campbell forgot the lyrics to his songs but could still play guitar solos. All the same, it's going to take more than music to deal humanely with the epidemic of dementia that threatens worldwide. Around 60,000 Kiwis are known to be affected (and many more cases go unreported), a figure predicted to almost triple by 2050.

Getting old is the greatest risk factor. Mum was relatively young when she got dementia in her early seventies; after 80, our chances increase to one in five, and after 90 to one in two. The problem is that our brains are wearing out before our bodies. What's more, they're so complex that an effective repair package is unlikely in my lifetime.

As more and more of us become eligible to receive the Queen's telegram, the equation's getting dangerously top-heavy: too few young and healthy, too many old and infirm. In a recent interview with Australian psycho-geriatric professor Henry Brodaty, broadcaster Kim Hill said it's hard to escape the conclusion medical science has enabled us to live too long. I expected Brodaty, who has studied Alzheimer's disease for 30 years, to at least fudge the issue. Instead he replied, 'That's absolutely right.'

Around this time, I had a dream that I went to get a bottle of wine but forgot where it was kept. I asked Megan if she knew, and she shouted that I couldn't remember anything, that I had to do something about it. I screamed back, making all sorts of excuses. Then Kate was hugging me. 'I can't bear it if I've got Alzheimer's, I just can't bear it,' I wept, burying my head in her chest.

'You can do better,' Pat said in the dream, which only convinced me something was wrong. I wondered if I'd have time to work out a new way of being before I lost my mind. I realised that Pat might not always be around to look after me, that I could be badly treated and no one would care.

If I do get dementia, I'd like to have the choice to say 'enough', for my sake and everyone else's. But coming up with rules that both empower and protect vulnerable people is fraught. For good reasons, assisted-dying protocols in places such as the Netherlands, Canada and the United States require a person to have a terminal illness, be of sound mind and give their free, informed consent when they're ready to die. The person often has to administer the lethal drug themselves or nominate somebody else at the time. People with advanced dementia can't do that.

Perhaps I could make the decision earlier and describe the conditions under which it should take effect. But until I'm in the thick of things, I'm not sure I can predict the tipping point when life won't seem worth living.

It doesn't seem fair to pass on that responsibility to a loved one either. How should they decide? When I can't talk? When I don't recognise them? When I stop responding to the headphones?

For the record, if it does comes down to the iPod, make it Mark Knopfler for me. In the car with Mum, I dispelled the gloomy conversation about medical intervention by turning up his jaunty little number about a quality shoe on the CD player. 'Pat says he's got a voice like a comfortable slipper,' I said.

Mum grinned. 'Who'd ever think of writing a song about shoes?'

I smiled at her and drummed the steering wheel with my fingers, then sang along with Mark about tired feet and sunny skies, rainy days and times when you'll be blue, all the way back to her place of incarceration.

CHAPTER TWENTY-TWO

THE STAR

MARIE, MUM'S SECOND new friend, also fell and broke her hip. Like Lesla, she was transferred to a public hospital and then back to the retirement village hospital wing. Mum didn't openly pine but a few days later Kate found her under the bed covers at two in the afternoon. 'I just want to get out of this place,' Mum shouted.

'So we did,' Kate emailed. 'Had a drive round the bays, then had the most lovely afternoon/evening in an armchair by the heater surrounded by 3 warm little bodies. They looked at schoolwork, awards, ebooks, photos, sculptures and watched *The Cat in the Hat* DVD. After a sizeable dinner and dessert, Sam and Andy showed her how to Google.' They looked up Mum's father, our father and the old hotel in Chamonix where Mum had stayed with Kate and Andy. 'She declined pain relief when I offered it but I gave her a couple of Panadol as she left,' Kate said.

Mum's bounce-back didn't last. Without a buddy, she floundered. 'I was quite taken aback at how anxious and unhappy she was when all her familiar faces were still out on the bus trip,'

Liz emailed after dropping her off at the village one afternoon. 'She wouldn't stay in the lounge with all the "resthomers". She wanted to wait in her room till the others were back.'

A bruise appeared on Mum's forehead; she had no idea how it had got there. Her left earlobe split into two flaps, as if she'd tugged an earring through it. The hairdresser had done it, she told Ginny, but hadn't charged Mum for the haircut. It didn't hurt but it looked strange. All we could do was suggest she grow her hair.

Mum's back pain flared up. When she walked, she leaned to the right and wobbled. We tried to make an appointment with the orthopaedic surgeon who'd diagnosed spondylolisthesis a few years earlier. After studying her x-rays, he said there was no point seeing her again. He suggested a walker and better pain relief.

When the walker arrived, Mum said it took up too much space in her studio and sent it back. When she remembered to use her walking stick, she'd leave it behind at her next stop. Everything disappeared: the tinea cream for her feet, the sensible shoes wide enough to accommodate her bunions, her cups, her mirror, her purse. Especially her purse. I'd search her room and swear it wasn't within its four walls, only for the next person to find it in her top drawer or down beside the bed. It was as if she had a secret panel that she spirited things behind and produced later just to make our heads spin.

Mum's heater worked, didn't work, worked again. After the exploding wheat bag destroyed her old microwave, we bought her a new one. Within weeks she'd blown it up again with another wheat bag that left a scorch mark across her carpet and stank out her room (and the whole corridor) for days.

Rose, in charge of snacks, couldn't keep up with the chocolate biscuits, cheese and crackers, nuts and wine that vanished from Mum's cupboard without her ever putting on an ounce. 'Let's not panic. We can do this, can't we?' she emailed, voicing our collective anxiety that Mum was coming off a plateau.

Mum turned down group outings and refused to go to the

Marsden Club. 'I think she's depressed,' Kate emailed. She'd found her in bed again, clutching the phone and our phone numbers, wearing the same clothes she'd had on for days.

We took to ringing her to see if she'd gone to the dining room. My heart sank one evening when she answered her studio phone at dinner time. Yes, she was hungry, she said, but her back was too sore to walk that far, and no one would give her Panadol without a doctor's prescription.

'You don't need a prescription for Panadol, Mum,' I said.

'Tell *them* that.'

I rang reception. The carer who'd tried to administer Mum's eye ointment answered. She said Mum had turned down dinner and refused to take Panadol while she was being watched. When I asked if she could take Mum something to eat now, she said all the food had gone.

Mum weighed 40 kilograms. It was 13 hours until breakfast and it was possible she'd missed lunch. It wasn't as if she could rustle herself up a snack later if she felt peckish. 'You must be able to give her something,' I said.

The carer agreed to make Mum a sandwich but was hesitant about offering her Panadol again. 'Your mother shouts at me,' she said. 'Every morning I have to go back with her pills ten times.'

'Please. Just try. She's in a lot of pain.'

'OK,' she said. 'Ring me back in half an hour to see how I got on.' I was glad she wanted to keep me informed, alarmed there seemed to be no support on site.

'*Ooh-la-la*,' Mum said when I let her know the carer was bringing her food.

'You have to be nice to her, Mum. She says she's scared of you.'

'Why?' Mum sounded incredulous.

'Might have something to do with the *ooh la las*.' I laughed and she joined in.

'I've never been rude to anyone in this place, Pip. Will she give me Panadol?'

'Yes, but you have to take it while she's watching.' There was a snort from the other end of the phone. 'It's the rules, Mum. There are some pretty dippy people in there who might hoard pills and take them all at once.'

'Well, you'd think they'd have learned to trust *me* by now.'

When I phoned the carer back, she sounded pleased with herself. She'd given Mum four club sandwiches and some grapes. 'Your mother took the Panadol like a lamb. You talked to her, didn't you?'

'Yes,' I said, relieved that Mum had remembered to cooperate, frustrated that I'd just spent another hour on the phone making sure she got fed, even if she was grumpy. For the zillionth time, I questioned the absence of strategies, staff supervision, team plans. The trouble with Mum's $395-a-week care package was that it came in units: meals offered, pills dispensed, showers supervised, activities and trips available. If she turned down any of the units, there seemed to be no holistic approach to her care. No one ever seemed to ask why Rosaleen might be anxious or angry or withdrawn, why she wouldn't eat or take her medication, and what might be done about it. There didn't even seem to be a system to pass on information from one shift to the next.

AT LABOUR WEEKEND, I met up with the women in my book to show them a draft. To my surprise, they asked me to read it aloud. There was silence as I recounted my version of the three years we'd lived and worked together in the Wellington gang scene. When we took a break, everyone avoided me.

That night, donning T-shirts with our Aroha Trust logo erased 30 years of hard-won maturity. By midnight the house looked like a train crash, drunken bodies staggering around and squaring up to fight over gang colours no one believed in any more. By morning most of the women had taken off or passed out. I spent the next day in shock, stunned by the power of the past to trigger old trauma.

As evening fell, Annie cooked roast lamb, the runaways returned, the sleepers emerged. I said they had to decide if they wanted a book. We sat in a circle. The first woman said no. Annie said she'd go along with everyone's wishes. Then one by one, all the other women said they did want their stories to be told. 'To break the cycle of silence and violence,' as one of them put it. What's more, they wanted to use their own names so they could speak out when the book was published.

If it was published, I reminded them.

It will be, their looks said.

I RANG MUM to invite her for lunch. She said she needed to stay where she was, that morning tea was a very good way to meet people and they always had a speaker. This was so out of character that I rang back later to invite her for tea. Again, she turned me down. I asked if she was all right. She said she was fine but she had to go. Her voice sounded a bit wired.

Next day, Rose overheard our favourite carer ask Mum if she wanted to lay a complaint. There'd been 'an incident', Rose learned. A resident who was known to shout and swear and wander had banged on Mum's door and gone into her room at one in the morning. When prompted, Mum said she'd woken up and been very scared. She didn't remember anything else. There'd been no staff in the area and no process to inform us. If the carer hadn't brought the matter up in front of Rose, we'd never have known. Mum's reluctance to leave the village the previous day made sense as a 'freeze' response in the face of danger.

The carer offered to help Mum write a letter of complaint.

We weren't looking for a scapegoat — wandering was inevitable and locking the studio doors at night carried other risks — but we did need to know our mother was safe. For some reason, we let the matter slide. By then, I fear, we'd lost faith in the studio management. Trying to get answers or action was like chasing mercury, especially with Mum as an unreliable witness. Calling the studios 'independent living' ignored the fact that residents couldn't look after themselves, otherwise they'd have been living in their own homes. A few had physical disabilities but most had dementia.

In a curious way, the facility manifested the symptoms of the disease it denied: confusion, inertia, forgetting to get back to us, denial and anger when challenged. The village GP seemed to us to be infected with the same malaise. 'Her medical file is a mess, he couldn't even find when she was last weighed,' Ginny emailed after Mum's three-monthly examination. 'But even he mentioned the poor nursing standards at the home, considering how well the group are doing financially, and how overworked the staff are.'

There's no doubt that Mum could be difficult. But if management had worked with us as a family, it might have made her life and their job easier. Instead we felt sidelined and troublesome when we stuck up for her. If we did ask staff to encourage Mum to change her clothes, or join in activities or eat, they'd tell her that her daughters said she must, sparking another round of outraged phone calls.

Some time after Mum died, I requested her care notes from the village. I read through them, searching for signs that the people who'd cared for her had cared about her. The village GP's initial assessment records Mum's medical history: 'dementia; falls — recurrent; gastro-oesophageal reflux; osteoporosis; gout'. Beside this list the word 'CONFABULATES!' is written in big letters with a box around it.

The Oxford English Dictionary told me it's a psychiatric term that means 'to fabricate imaginary experiences as compensation for loss of memory'. Other sources said it was common in dementia and stressed the person had no intention to deceive. Which was why the capitals and the exclamation mark troubled me — as if suggesting that Mum's skewed reality was humorous or surprising or deliberate.

The GP's jottings at Mum's subsequent three-monthly medical checks are minimal. So are the staff notes during Mum's 26-month studio stay: just 10 A4 lined sheets, almost half in the first six weeks before she'd committed to buy. There are 70 entries in all. Around a third record Mum's refusal to shower or eat or take her pills; there's no sense of a broad plan for her care; few of the comments convey understanding about her mental state.

Two entries stamped with 'V Coordinator visit', stand out: 'A very pleasant lady with a great sense of humour,' says the first, a month after Mum moved in. A week later, a second entry describes meeting Mum on the wrong floor, heading towards the hospital, not for the first time. The coordinator says she took Mum to the lift and showed her the star beside the button for her own floor. 'I said she was "a star" and I'll keep calling her that to try and trigger her memory.'

I imagine Mum's face lighting up at the compliment. I wish I could thank the coordinator for her humanity.

CHAPTER TWENTY-THREE

HOLE IN THE HALLWAY

MUM COULD STILL recite the first and last names of the 29 children in her primary school photo, although when she came to the pretty young girl with the bow in her hair and the level gaze in the middle of the middle row, she said 'Rosaleen Waigth' as if she was simply another classmate.

Mum's short-term memory was almost completely gone. Sometimes, though, she still surprised us. In May 2008 I made a list of things she'd recently remembered: to be nice to the carer who'd brought her sandwiches and Panadol; that Rose's new house in Seatoun had all those steps but a stunning harbour view; the name of the jeweller who'd made her wedding ring; the surname of the accountant who'd managed her money.

Reading this list made me think about the act of remembering — and forgetting. All of us forget things all the time. Our imperfect memories are magnificent filters that stop us drowning in detail and being overwhelmed by the past. It's not so much time that's a great healer as *forgetting,* which takes the edge off even the saddest and most traumatic events so we can get on with our lives.

Which memories we keep and which we discard happens unconsciously. In spite of Mum's faulty mechanism, her list suggests she remembered things for the same reasons as the rest of us: self-interest (the sandwiches and Panadol); danger (Rose's steps); life-changing events (her wedding ring); survival (money).

Even without dementia, the playing field's not level. Some people have photographic memories, memories like elephants, specialised memories for faces, names or numbers. My own feels more like Martha Gellhorn's. In *Travels with Myself and Another,* Gellhorn said she thinks she was born with a weak memory, 'as one can be born with a weak heart or weak ankles'. This admission from one of the twentieth century's top war correspondents gives me comfort. When I was young, I could inhale information, regurgitate it for exams and promptly forget it. As I age, even that skill's fading. To borrow Gellhorn's words, 'I forget places, people, events, and books as fast as I read them. All the magnificent scenery, the greatest joy of travel, blurs. As to dates — What year? What month? — the situation is hopeless.'

Gellhorn said she was 'still waiting for the promised time, said to arrive with advancing age, when you forget what you ate for breakfast but the past becomes brilliantly clear, like a personal *son et lumière.*'

That didn't happen to Mum. It's true that in the early stages of dementia, she spoke more often and openly about the past, but that was because she let her guard down, I think, not because her memories lit up. Later, old photos and a small stock of stories provided vital anchors in her crumbling world. But the stories became fuzzier, not brighter, and she didn't seem to spend much time consorting with ghosts.

Not consciously at least. When I emailed my siblings to say her angry phone calls were driving me crazy again, Matt replied, 'Oh dear, Pip, something that happened in the mists of memory has definitely wired the familial brain for you to be the fall guy.'

In desperation, I asked if I could replace my phone number at the top of Mum's list with Liz's in the hope that Mum might think twice about making toll calls. Rose replied that she'd considered taking my name off the list altogether. But the prospect made me feel even more desolate. All I could see was the empty space on the list and a matching hole in Mum's heart. If she didn't have my phone number, I might cease to exist for her at all.

When Mum's agitation continued, Liz asked her friend, a geriatrician, if we should add an anti-depressant or anti-psychotic to her cocktail of drugs, as someone had suggested. But he said Risperidone upped the risk of stroke, while anti-depressants increased drowsiness and the risk of falls and were less effective for people with dementia. 'He said people in rest homes often get treated for the staff's symptoms rather than their own when the best meds would be a cup of tea and a chat!' Liz emailed.

MATT WHISTLED INTO town again. We were too frazzled to quiz him much about life in Hanoi or Myanmar or Bangkok, and welcomed him as another pair of hands. But he only went to see Mum a few times and seemed oblivious to her insatiable need for company.

After he left, Ginny emailed the sisters her disappointment in his efforts. I agreed with her. But Liz came to his defence. 'I actually think it might be easier being in the rest home groove when you're doing it often,' she replied. 'I think when you come back infrequently it seems like such an "event" and especially without his own transport it's probably just "too hard" when he's only got a couple of weeks. Oh well, I'm probably excusing my own contribution there too, which is paltry compared with yours.'

This wasn't true. Liz was constantly making the four-hour drive from Hastings, phoning Mum, looking after her affairs from afar, buoying up the rest of us. I didn't envy her being outside the daily fray, always feeling torn and guilty. I didn't envy Matt either, living in two worlds, arriving home to our exhaustion and demands and female ways when what he needed was a holiday.

Apart from her children, only a handful of people kept in touch with Mum. She drove some of them away. In the end I advised her most loyal friend to stop going to see her; something about her triggered Mum's scathing, pitiless side. We didn't have the energy to deal with the friend's hurt feelings after each visit; I was hardly able to deal with my own.

As the weeks went by, I noticed less anger in Mum's calls, more sadness and anxiety. What day was it? Did I have her weekly schedule? Would there be morning tea?

One afternoon she rang to say it was happy hour at the bar. Would I go over and have a drink with her? If I have one regret during this time, it's that I didn't jump in the car that grey afternoon and race across town to keep her company. I didn't even soften the blow with therapeutic fibbing ('I'd love to, Mum, I'm on my way.') I couldn't bear the thought of her sitting on her bed with her purse, waiting, waiting, waiting for me to show up. Instead, I told her the truth: that by the time I got through peak hour traffic, happy hour would be over.

Only it wasn't the whole truth. What I didn't say was that I hated spending time in the place where I expected her to be happy. On our days together, I'd whip in, pick her up and take her back to my world. I told myself I was doing it for her sake — she loved getting out and being with family.

But I was also doing it for myself. I couldn't face the sterile surroundings, the loopy conversation, the pall of confusion and boredom that enveloped the residents, knowing that no matter how long I stayed, it would never be long enough. Now I think

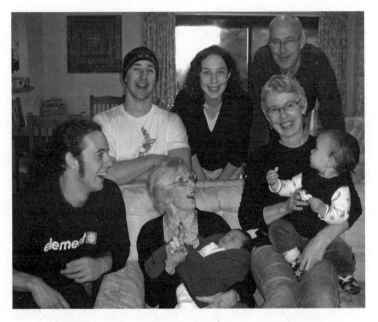

Mum, the matriarch of four generations, and my family on her seventy-seventh birthday, 18 November 2006, soon after she moved into the retirement village. Back, from left: Liam, Megan, Pat. Front: Jackson, Mum holding three-day-old Avah, me holding Rome.

how heroic Mum was, living each day with dementia swirling all around her as well as inside her head.

Kate did better when she rang Mum 'and got the full outpouring: the back pain, the nausea, everybody gone for the weekend. Couldn't possibly walk, couldn't possibly eat, what was the point of it all? I commiserated, and then gently pointed out that if she wasn't able to stay independent and get herself to meals then she wouldn't be allowed to stay in her nice little studio. She went very quiet, then, "Please could you come in and have lunch with me?" she asked. (How telling is that?)'

So Kate did. 'We sorted clothes, went through papers and did a general tidy. Over the next 5 minutes she asked me 5 times if I would have lunch with her. We ambled happily down to lunch. She couldn't remember where she sat and one of the staff set her off in the wrong direction. Another yelled out she was going the wrong way. I gently explained to them both how lost Mum was without Marie, how it had affected her confidence and state of mind — please could they ensure she sat with people she knew. (I swear I saw one roll her eyes as I was talking.)'

Kate was angry. 'I'd love to set up a day course for those nurses where they were plonked in a place where they didn't know the layout, the ground rules, what they were meant to be doing and then got told off for doing the wrong thing. It might engender some empathy.'

We requested another meeting with management. They agreed Mum had deteriorated and was missing Marie, though they denied she ever stayed in her room all day and said if she skipped meals she'd always be given food. We asked them to report back to us in two weeks. If nothing else, they knew we were watching.

Afterwards, I took Mum to a café for lunch. As she tucked into a piece of quiche, she complained about the guitarist crooning into a microphone a few feet away. I half expected her to put her fingers in her ears like the toddler at the next table.

Back in her studio, I moisturised her cracked heels and crooked toes that were plagued with a fungal infection in spite of regular trips to the podiatrist.

'That's lovely,' she murmured. 'I could let you do that forever.'

'I DON'T GO out at night,' said Mum as she teetered on our front door step.

Tonight you do, I thought, kneeling beside her and trying to guide her right foot down onto the porch as she clung to the door jamb. Beyond her, the wind whipped the power lines and misty rain danced in the halo of the street light. 'Just one step, Mum, that's all,' I said, thinking of Liz's observation that taking that one step was as big a deal for Mum as bungee jumping would be for us.

Too bad. I'd booked tickets to the documentary *Young at Heart.* We were going and that was that. It took 10 minutes to cover the five metres from door to porch, porch to path, path to gate, gate to car. Me behind, holding Mum steady as she inched along the fence, Pat in front with an umbrella to keep her dry. I blanked out how I was going to manage at the other end.

The cinema glowed like a lighthouse in the storm. Pat helped me get Mum out of the car and, with a concerned look, went off to find a park. Mum clutched my arm while I picked up our tickets in the mercifully empty foyer. Thankfully, the movie was screening in a ground floor theatre. As we started along the corridor, Mum let go of me and strode on ahead. Inside, she handled the shallow steps with ease, and by the time Pat arrived with ice creams, we were settled in our seats. He looked astonished. 'I thought I was going to have to carry her in,' he whispered in my ear.

That's the trouble with vascular dementia. It affected Mum's balance, strength and spatial sense — but only sometimes. When she felt safe, she could still walk stiffly but unaided. Outside she became paralysed. Her body could do it; it was her mind that was unreliable. How unreliable I only considered after reading *Still Alice,* Lisa Genova's novel about a woman who has early onset Alzheimer's disease. Alice imagines a hole in her hallway floor that prevents her going out the front door. All those times Mum refused to put one foot in front of the other, it never occurred to me to ask her what she saw.

The film, about a group of Massachusetts senior citizens who form a choir, was worth the effort. My favourite choir member was Eileen, 93, who had her own key to the rest home because she got back from choir practice after the staff had gone to bed. There was nothing saccharine about the story. Two lead characters died during the making of it and, at the final concert, 83-year-old Fred sang with breathing tubes through his nose and a portable oxygen tank at his feet.

Nevertheless, an abyss separated Mum, engrossed beside me, from the choir members. No matter how sick or disabled, they could pick up melodies and harmonies, adapt old songs to new rhythms, learn their lines. By the time we got back to the car, Mum wouldn't know she'd been to a movie, and the only Fred she'd recall would be her husband — although I had to believe the experience had nourished her spirit in some way, just as a book whose plot I've forgotten may have nourished mine.

Mum's failing memory wasn't the saddest thing, though. Watching the choir members interact with their charismatic choirmaster, resolve tensions and put the group's needs before their own brought home to me Mum's loss of awareness, not only of herself but also of others. Dementia had stolen her ability to walk a mile in someone else's shoes, a gulf as impassable as the hole Alice saw in her hallway.

That was the saddest thing.

CHAPTER TWENTY-FOUR

TOOTHACHE

ONE DAY MUM opened her mouth and there was a gap where her top front tooth should have been. The crown had fallen out without her noticing. I phoned a dental practice close by and told the receptionist Mum was very frail. She assured me there was parking and walk-on access to the first-floor surgery. Mum and I arrived in a September squall to find a poky carpark chock-a-block with builders' gear. I double-parked in front of a plasterer's van, and steered her through mounds of rubble towards a steep outside ramp, the access I'd been promised.

Mum clutched the handrail and shuffled up the slippery ramp as if her feet were bound. Next time, I vowed, I'd organise a walker, no matter how much she protested. At the top was a heavy swing door that opened onto us. I got her through it and under cover. Two more swing doors lay between us and the dentist's surgery. By the time we got to the waiting room, Mum was shivering with cold and fear. I sat her down, glared at the receptionist and went to sort out the car.

In the dentist's chair, Mum panicked when he tipped her backwards. She panicked again when he tried to insert a bite-blocker into her mouth to take x-rays. It hurt, she said, flailing her hands in front of her mouth. And she couldn't breathe.

The dentist's nurse stroked Mum's arm and talked to her softly.

'She has dementia,' I said under my breath.

Mum unclenched her teeth. 'What did you say?'

'I said you have a denture.' It was my finest moment of therapeutic fibbing.

The dentist succeeded in x-raying the trouble spot, then gave up trying to examine the rest of Mum's mouth. He said he couldn't restore the crown or attach another tooth to her bottom denture; he'd have to make a separate one. I had no idea how she'd learn to insert it but gave him the go-ahead: we couldn't leave her looking like Fagin.

Three appointments and more than $1000 later, the denture was ready. It'd be a bit tight for a week or so until she got used to it, the dentist said. But Mum couldn't think in terms of a week or so. If something wasn't right, she wanted it gone NOW.

The denture joined a long list of things to be misplaced. 'Pleased to report we found it in the little crystal dish on her dresser,' Rose emailed. 'Sad to report that Mum can't stand it and despite my best efforts and lots of patience and instruction (so difficult to work out which way round, top from bottom and so on), as soon as it was in her mouth she felt she was choking and was desperate to get it out again. Commented about the terrible dentist and the need to look for another. I offered that she doesn't have to wear it if she's OK with the gap. Well, she's not — but she doesn't want to wear it. Upshot is that the denture is wrapped in a tissue and now rests in the other, empty crystal dish on the dresser.'

That afternoon Rose took Mum, minus tooth, to Marie's funeral. Like Lesla, Mum's second new friend lived only a few months after breaking her hip. At the funeral Rose learned of Marie's long association with Māori cultural club Ngāti Pōneke, a connection we'd never have guessed: dementia wipes a person's history as cleanly as a duster on a blackboard.

'She was welcomed into the church with a karakia and 3 older Pākehā women sang a song in Māori in her honour,' Rose emailed. 'Pretty impressive for an 88-year-old!' Rose also met Marie's relations for the first time. 'They appeared to be a strong-minded and direct extended family who had grown up together and knew each other well. There was genuine fondness for Marie, but most of it in the past.'

Afterwards, Rose and her son Tom took Mum out for lunch. 'It seems to me she has lost most of her capability of being attentive and absorbing information — but still feels very connected to us all at an intuitive level,' Rose said. 'She was philosophical over Marie's death and said, "It happens to us all, Rose." She didn't have a lot to say to Tom, but all the way home repeated what a nice boy Tom is — so very gentle. (Of course, I agree!)'

A week later Mum's new denture vanished, never to be seen again. I pictured her burying it in a pot plant or flushing it down the loo with a satisfying *whoosh*. There was no point going through the palaver of getting another one made. Mum forgot the tooth was missing and we resigned ourselves to her rakish grin.

Others were less understanding. The daughter of a resident took me aside and told me my mother was such a lady; she'd be mortified if she realised how she looked — as if that hadn't occurred to us. Then a carer told us other residents were picking on Mum, partly because of her toothless gap. This was more worrying. But believe me, if we'd known how to get a tooth into Mum's mouth and make it stay there, we would have.

AS CHRISTMAS APPROACHED, I conducted my annual test of Mum's skill level by getting her to help me make mince pies.

I was surprised to find she could do everything she'd done two years earlier: grease the patty pans, fill the pastry cases with fruit mince, put the tops on and prick them with a fork. But when I turned away, she piled more filling on top of the tops and after we'd put the first dozen in the oven, she lost interest.

Reluctantly I took her to the Marsden Club Christmas party at The Pines, a function centre perched above Wellington's south coast. Floor-to-ceiling windows overlooked a blur of sea and sky as bleak as I felt myself. My Christmas Grinch sneered at the smiling helpers and the tables laden with food. I wanted to run away: from the noise and small talk, the wheelchairs and walkers, the bent bodies and listless eyes. Mum looked like she wanted to run away too.

At lunch we sat next to a woman and her older husband who had Alzheimer's disease. She'd recently had to put him in a rest home, she said. Although she spent all day with him, every morning began with a distressed phone call from him begging to go home.

I'd often wished Dad had been alive to look after Mum when she got dementia. Now I felt grateful their relationship had been spared that heartbreak. If it was difficult for us to put Mum into care, how much harder it must be to send your soulmate away. I wondered if it'd be worse to be the person making the morning phone call or the one receiving it.

A year later, I got an inkling. At my friend Petra's house, I got up to make a cup of tea; we were doing some work together. I filled her round kettle, put it on the stove, turned on the gas and walked away. When I came back a minute later, flames were licking the sides of the kettle and the base was melting over the element like a Dali pocket watch. The kettle was electric. Mortified, I spent the next hour chipping black plastic off the pristine stovetop. Never mind, Petra said, when I offered to buy her a new kettle. She had another one just like it.

A few days later, she asked me to make another cup of tea.

'I'm surprised you'll let me,' I laughed. I got up, took the kettle off its stand, filled it, put it on the stove and turned on the gas. Then she was beside me, her hand on my shoulder, her voice unbearably gentle: 'It doesn't go on the stove, remember.'

I was devastated. I could (almost) rationalise doing it once. Petra used to have a round kettle that did go on the gas stove, and the first time it had been sitting on the bench, not its stand. But nothing could justify doing it twice, especially when I'd just made a joke about it. Nothing except early onset Alzheimer's.

In the days that followed, I watched myself intently. When a familiar word hovered just beyond my grasp, when I wandered off with someone else's supermarket trolley, when I aimed the car remote control at the front door of our house, my stomach churned. There and then, I made a pact with the devil. Give me physical pain, I begged, but don't rob me of my mind.

This was not a completely uninformed bargain. Ever since my kids were young, I'd had chronic pain that drilled between my shoulder blades, burned at the base of my spine, gnawed in places I hadn't known were there. On bad days, nothing else mattered. But however hopeless or helpless the pain made me feel, I had my mind to seek comfort and healing. If I had dementia I'd be at its mercy, as would my aching muscles and joints.

After the kettle incidents I got rid of my aluminium stock pot, swallowed fish oil tablets and tormented myself with Sudoku puzzles. I did one other thing too: I threw out the Nortriptyline pills I'd been taking for two years for chronic pain. My mind seemed to clear. Some time later I asked a pain specialist whether the drug could have made me disoriented. Yes, he said, it did create changes in the brain. Were those changes reversible when you stopped taking it, I asked? Not necessarily, he said.

The spectre of dementia still hangs over me. A German study that shows Alzheimer's disease can be predicted decades in advance by people's ability to navigate through a virtual maze makes my knees tremble. I've always been absentminded; getting lost is my speciality. 'Don't worry, it makes me feel useful,' says Pat as he reins me in yet again. But I do worry.

My sisters worry about themselves too, I think. We're not alone. Most New Zealanders know someone with dementia and a quarter of us have been involved in their direct care and support. Seeing what it does to loved ones makes many people fear the disease more than cancer.

Pat asks me why I care so much if I do get it. It's a good question; he clearly doesn't. When I'm honest, shame is high on the list. For being foolish and dithery. For not being in control. For being an oddity and a burden. I dread the frustration and disappointment and isolation. Beneath that is a horror of being slowly stripped of everything I love and think I am. The Buddhists are no doubt right when they say my personality's just an illusion — but try telling my ego that.

Of course, Mum weighs heavily on my mind, although having a parent with the disease doesn't increase your own risk much, except in one rare form. Nor are the possible triggers in her life repeated in mine.

Mum's high blood pressure was the immediate cause of the mini-strokes that led to vascular dementia; my own blood pressure has always been low. Mum had to leave home at 13 to go to boarding school; I left at 19 of my own accord. Mum had six kids, four in quick succession, with an absent husband and little family support; I have three children who grew up near their grandparents, and all those sisters to back me up. Mum endured Dad's epilepsy and became his caregiver in middle age; Pat has stayed healthy and looks after me. Mum lived in an age when women were expected to suppress their needs and desires; I've enjoyed unprecedented freedom and opportunity.

There are some things I can do to improve my chances. Scientists have discovered that our remarkable brains — which weigh about the same as a thin laptop and are infinitely more complex — can change and heal in response to mental experience, a process known as neuroplasticity. The circuitry's so interconnected that if we lose one neural pathway, another may fire up. It is possible to teach an old brain new tricks.

Christine Bryden — the Australian advocate who showed me some people with dementia have insight — has defied medical science by living a full life for 20 years after being diagnosed with early onset Alzheimer's disease, although in scans her brain looks like it's been nibbled by mice. Seven years after I heard her speak in Wellington, Christine wrote a memoir, *Before I Forget*. In it she raises the possibility that her high 'cognitive reserve' — the extra brain capacity she inherited at birth or developed as a child from her mother's intellectual stimulation — has helped slow the disease.

We need to future-proof our own children, she says, by keeping their brain cells active and connected. Not that there are any guarantees of success. While some of Christine's fellow activists also remain high-functioning, others equally intelligent and able have succumbed quickly to the disease.

Christine's memoir makes me wonder if Mum's genes and upbringing shored up her competence as she lost brain power. She'd told me her father had a very good memory. 'What he read, he remembered. He was a fount of knowledge. He could answer your questions.'

There was nothing John Henry Waigth couldn't do, it seems. He was as practical as he was visionary, wiring the family's Roxburgh house himself and powering it with a generator before lobbying for electricity for the district. On top of his business, church and political interests, he gardened, taught himself accounting and how to play the piano, kept meticulous weather records and built an aviary in his backyard.

For Christmas when Mum was 11, her father gave her two hard-covered tomes. *The Story of the World* and *Our Generation: A Pictorial Record of Britain in Our Own Times* encouraged his daughter to set her sights beyond the small rural town of her birth, even if they still focused on the achievements of men and the motherland.

John Harry, in turn, could have his grandmother to thank for his high cognitive reserve. Catherine Brown — she of the three husbands — may have been illiterate: she signed her marriage certificate with an 'X'. But she had the foresight to include school books in the limited possessions she brought to Roxburgh East by pack horse, and was instrumental in setting up the first school there in 1864. John Harry's father was one of three initial pupils.

Studies show that education can push out the onset and progression of dementia. So can a healthy lifestyle: good food, exercise, social connections, a positive attitude. We might not be able to prevent or cure the disease, says New Zealand professor Richard Faull, director of the Centre for Brain Research, but if we can delay it by five years across the board, we can halve its incidence and improve people's quality of life while they die of other things first.

When it comes to preparing for the future, Mum's emotional turmoil also convinces me of the need to befriend my shadow side. If I don't get dementia, this still seems like my best chance at a good life. And if Sally Magnusson and Gabor Maté are right that repressed emotions can trigger the disease, the sooner I face my own demons, the better. Even if they don't cause the disease, chances are they'd sabotage my civilised veneer if I got it.

If all that fails, I can only hope that the people who love me will continue to show up when I can't. Look in any retirement village, rest home or dementia unit and you'll see what a big ask that is.

WHEN LIZ SUGGESTED having Mum to stay in Hastings for a week over Christmas, we leapt at the offer. Mum hadn't spent a night away from her studio in two years. But we figured the upheaval couldn't be worse than the heightened loneliness she felt at this time of year; it was a good chance for Liz to observe her closely and might clarify our concerns about her ongoing care.

A few days into Mum's visit, Liz emailed, 'Mum's happy and I haven't gone mad. I started writing the answers to the most frequently asked questions on labels and sticking them on her sleeves so when I was asked "Is this your room?" or "So how did I get here?" I could just point to the relevant label which saved my voice and reduced Mum to a fit of giggles. The only bad day was when we had a couple of friends over and Mum turned into a witch. However, so long as she had company and wasn't stressed or being asked to do something she didn't want to do, she was as sweet as a lamb.'

Liz discovered that while Mum always knew her name, she didn't always know their relationship. Looking at family photos on Liz's wall, Mum would say, 'So how are you related to these people?' or 'What was your family name?' When Liz explained, Mum would say, 'Well, isn't it a small world!' and once, 'It's very confusing having two Lizs!' Liz wondered if the change of scene had thrown Mum or if she'd been better able to hide her confusion among us all.

In an update on New Year's Day, 24 hours before Mum was due to return to her studio, Liz reported, 'Mum is very happy and settled (too settled?). I took her to get her hair done yesterday and overheard the hairdresser asking her how long she was staying on in Hawke's Bay. Her reply: "Forever". Oh, dear.'

CHAPTER TWENTY-FIVE

ALONE IS LONELY

From: Liz
To: Rose; Ginny; Pip; Kate; Matt
Sent: Friday, Jan 2, 2009 07:00 PM
Subject: Oh dear Mamma Mia

Damn. Damn. Damn!
Last night Mum fell and hurt her shoulder. I'd put her to bed a short while earlier expecting her to sleep through, as she had every other night. (I've been sleeping outside her door so I know she can snore for 10 hrs.)

Luckily Dave and I were having a cup of tea in the next room and heard something because she didn't cry out and I found her sitting on the floor at the end of the bed. Weirdly there were magazines strewn all over the bed so she'd had a busy 10 minutes or so after lights out. It kind of bugs me, as the nights had been so settled, but I guess we'll never know.

Mum says she bent down to pick up a tissue, but anyway, she's still heavy enough to have broken the head of her humerus. It's an impacted fracture, which is apparently the best kind as it doesn't require surgery but of course it's v painful and she can't use her left arm which has implications which are . . . enormous . . . e.g. just getting her to stand up from sitting is taking all my and Dave's ingenuity, persuasion and sometimes, as a last resort, brute force. I'd given her a shower or bath every day but how to do this now, I'm not sure. Also toileting, which she has needed help with more than once, is going to be trickier with this new disability.

So sorry to be sending this kind of progress report. I'm not sure where to from here. I think Mum should stay on at least for another week or so — the Dr says 2 weeks healing but that seems optimistic to me, but we could just see how it goes. She certainly can't go back to her studio like this, so it's going to mean tough decisions if she doesn't get back to 'independent living' ability. Any suggestions or ideas will be gratefully received of course.

So, how's your year been so far? :)

xx Liz

My year had been looking good. Random House had accepted my book and it was coming out in July. Mum kept saying it was going to solve all her Christmas present problems although it'd be a bit late for that. I'd been checking my emails to see if the proofreader had been in touch when I saw Liz's message.

Mum kept telling Liz, 'Thank goodness it's not my good arm.' Sadly, this wasn't true. Her old rotator cuff injury meant she couldn't lift a cup of tea to her mouth with her right arm. Now she couldn't use the left one at all.

Rose alerted the retirement village to Mum's fall, to be told it was in lock-down after another norovirus outbreak. Even if she'd been well, Mum couldn't go back to her studio for at least a week. We wondered when they'd planned to let us know or if they'd have waited until she turned up at the door.

Liz, with help from Dave and her kids who were home for Christmas, seemed composed at the prospect of Mum's extended stay, even when Mum announced she'd received a letter from a woman thanking her for selling her studio. Liz arranged for home help in the form of 'a large, cheerful lady with prominent front teeth, a bad back and shortness of breath' who received the same withering reception from Mum as the carers at Colville Street.

More popular was an André Rieu DVD that Liz had picked up from The Warehouse. 'I don't know if it's André or the old songs or the waltzes or maybe it's all the crowd shots of happy pensioners but something about it engages Mum like no other TV she watches,' Liz said. 'She also loves *The Three Tenors Christmas Special*.'

The downstairs bedroom where Mum slept had two exits. Liz camped outside one but woke in the early hours to find that Mum — who needed help with everything — had steered the walker to the bathroom through the other, put her incontinence pad in the rubbish bin, left the walker behind and gone back to bed unaided.

'If I hadn't seen it with my own eyes, I wouldn't have believed it,' Liz said. 'It reminds me of that fairy story where the elves come out at night.' It was only later she realised that Mum was operating on auto-pilot because she was half-asleep. 'The fear arises when she is awake and aware; that's what paralyses her, not her physical disability.'

Anxious that Mum might fall again, Liz mused that she might lie on the floor so that Mum stepped on her if she got out of bed. 'But she'd probably manage to crawl out the other side. I will have to do something though — Dave thinks we should tie a bell on to her.'

'Thanks for looking after Tinkerbell and maintaining your sense of humour, Liz,' Ginny replied.

Beneath Liz's whimsy were hints about how exhausting Mum's care had become. 'Mum hates EVER to be alone,' Liz said. 'She NEVER wants to lie on her bed or go to her bedroom during the day. Her book and her stick are her 2 daytime anchors — both utterly useless as far as their original purpose goes, but both invaluable security. I've put some photos inside her book which she shuffles through endlessly. In her bedroom, the fluffy rug and her pillow are her two night-time anchors (phew, Kate!) She does seem to go through an anxiety slump in the mid-late afternoon. I wonder if there's a village circadian rhythm at play here — maybe there's a regular downtime in the afternoons when there aren't activities or something, or is it anxiety about dinner time?'

Liz was describing a syndrome called *sundowning* that affects people with dementia, although we didn't know that then. Mum's fall had sent her tumbling a few more rungs down the ladder. By the time Pat and I turned up to help a week later, she seemed to have folded into herself, although she greeted me kindly and reserved her sharp tongue for Liz, who'd replaced me in the front line.

My sister was a natural nurse, calm and gentle, with the authoritative air of an eldest daughter. I marvelled at the systems she'd set up and was happy to assume helper status in the bathroom as she sponged Mum's emaciated frame. Mum stood regal and resigned, her breasts scalloped against her chest, her left arm and shoulder mottled with purple-yellow bruising. There was a gaunt, dignified beauty about her, an ease in her nakedness I'd never seen before and wanted to applaud — or perhaps it was just indifference, a vacating of her body along with her mind.

As Mum clung to me, Liz knelt and guided her feet into her pyjama legs. But no matter how hard Liz tugged, the pyjamas wouldn't rise above Mum's calves.

Finally in her haughtiest voice, Mum announced, 'My legs are both in the same hole.' She paused. 'If that's not being too par-*tic*-u-lar.' She glared at me and I tried to keep a straight face while below me Liz's shoulders shook with silent laughter.

It was a rare light moment. By the time we got Mum into bed, we were too exhausted to do anything but head there ourselves. Especially Liz, who'd been on night duty for two weeks, jumping at every sound on the other side of the door. Each day felt as daunting as scaling Mount Everest. When Mum woke, she'd be dazed and sluggish. It took hours to get her up and dressed and give her breakfast: a teaspoonful of melon and banana chopped into tiny pieces, a few sips of tea through a straw. Since her fall, anything starchy or stringy got stuck in her teeth and throat, rolled around in her mouth and spat out into the tissues she kept up her sleeve. It was hard to persuade her to eat at all.

At least the morning ritual provided a focus. After that the hours stretched ahead like a trek up the North Face. Mum spent most of her day sitting in the TV room. She never wanted to be alone; her need for us had become as constant as her need for air.

We took it in turns to sit with her. She couldn't talk much but complained if we picked up a magazine or tuned into the one-day cricket. I tried to read her Joe Bennett's hitch-hiking adventures around New Zealand from *A Land of Two Halves.* The first time she loved the descriptions of old haunts like Geraldine and Dunedin; the second time, she became fretful. André Rieu's magic wore off.

Sometimes Mum was sweet. Sometimes she'd sit with a faraway look and I'd want to draw her wasted body to mine and kiss away her terrors. If she dozed in her armchair, one eye would open at any attempt by us to creep out of the room or hold a whispered conversation. As she shuffled through her photos she'd say, 'Do my family know where I am? I feel like I've just been dumped here.'

Pat did his best to help but Mum needed her daughters. When

I realised she'd emptied her bowels one morning, I wanted to shout for Liz and flee, as I'd done with my grandmother when I was 13. This time I forced myself to clean her. It wasn't so bad. As I patted the papery skin dry on legs that seemed too thin to hold her up, Mum asked me how we were related.

In spite of Liz's forewarning, a small jolt went through my heart. 'I'm your daughter,' I said.

Mum scanned my face. 'That means I must be ancient,' she said with a wry smile.

IN THE AFTERNOONS, we'd push Mum around the block in a wheelchair borrowed from the hospital, trying to dispel her lethargy with bright chat about other people's gardens while Liz's miniature Schnauzer, Ellie, strained on her leash. One day I took Mum outside and sat her in the shade, overlooking Liz's well-kept lawn. The air hummed with cicadas. To our left lay the unruffled swimming pool where our kids had splashed and dived and vied with their cousins on hot summer days such as this.

As I stood behind her brushing her fine, white hair, I murmured in her ear, then realised I was breathing on her neck. 'Sorry,' I said.

'No,' she said. 'I like it. It makes me feel I'm not alone.' She bent down to pat Ellie. Mum and I were both nervous around animals but the little dog's quizzical expression and boxy beard disarmed us. Ellie got up and hared around the lawn chasing white butterflies. She stopped, flipped onto her back, rolled her plump body in the grass and waved her paws in the air, then tore after the butterflies again.

'Look at Ellie,' Mum said in an awed tone. 'She's alone but she's not lonely.' Of all the things dementia had stolen from her, it may have been the loss of self-sufficiency she felt most keenly. Trapped in the present moment, unable to remember the past or anticipate the future, she needed other people to anchor her. To be alone *was* to be lonely.

Being imprisoned in the here-and-now had one advantage: it worked wonders for Mum's broken shoulder. If it hurt, it hurt; if it didn't, she forgot it was injured. She didn't contract around the memory of pain or worry it might come back, as I did with mine. In other words, she didn't add the useless layer of suffering generated by the mind that the Buddhists call dukkha. Despite her disdain for both the sling she was meant to wear and the recommended exercises, her shoulder began to heal.

The same could not be said for the rest of her. After two days of barely eating or drinking, Mum's speech was slurred and she was weak and confused. Liz made an appointment with a GP. It took us so long to get Mum into the car that we considered asking him to come out to the carpark to examine her. In the end, we put one arm through each of hers and dragged her inside like a rag doll, her feet skimming the ground. As we sat in the waiting room, her head lifted off her chest, a glint came into her eyes, a small red circle appeared on each cheek. By the time the GP called her into his office, she could walk by herself.

'So you've had an accident,' he said in that jocular way people reserve for the elderly and children.

'No,' said Mum, in vowels as clipped as the queen's. 'I did it on purpose.'

It was impossible to explain how low she'd been. We took her home.

Next day she was worse, unable to talk or swallow her pills. This time the GP came to us. He suggested a drip to rehydrate her but that would mean a trip to hospital: needles and tubes and strangers. We couldn't bring ourselves to put her through it, knowing how upset she'd be.

Meanwhile the Wellington sisters put Mum's name on the waiting list of an aged-care facility in Newtown that we'd heard good things about. The retirement village was still battling norovirus and was reluctant to take Mum back without a full health assessment to determine her level of care. This put us in a Catch-22 situation. The assessment could only be done in Wellington by Mum's district health board, but Mum couldn't go back to Wellington until she'd been assessed. 'TGFS' (Thank God for sisters), Rose signed off in an email outlining all this and setting up yet another meeting with Ginny and Kate.

At the end of Liz's street was a rest home called Gracelands. Liz and I took it in turns to check it out. Although Mum would have to share an en suite, the residents' rooms were light, twice as big as any we'd seen in Wellington, and set in gorgeous grounds. The manager said all the right things about the care Mum would get and offered to take her at once, probably due to Dave's standing in the Hawke's Bay medical community. We accepted, then rang the others. They balked at the prospect of living 200 miles from Mum and questioned the load on Liz. But no one had a better plan.

We kept the news from Mum. But as I was cooking tea, she walked into the kitchen without help and began arguing about why she had to stay in Hastings and why we'd made her sell Colville Street. At dinner, she downed a small bowl of stewed apple and ice cream, the most food she'd eaten in days. Afterwards, she talked about Roxburgh. Then she took herself to the toilet and swallowed two Panadol and a sleeping pill without a hitch. The fight-back was on.

Next morning she was awake early, unusually alert. As we fed and dressed her, Liz and I were close to tears. We'd chosen Gracelands for the comatose mother who couldn't walk or eat, not this keyed-up, astute mother who wouldn't let us out of her sight.

Dave beckoned us into his office and closed the door. 'You don't have to do this, you know,' he said.

I thought of his efforts to secure the room in the rest home, of the helpful manager who'd fast-tracked Mum's admission and was waiting for us to arrive.

'It doesn't matter,' he said. 'If you want to change your mind, I'll let her know she's not coming.'

Our resolve evaporated. One predicament replaced another. I toyed with the idea of staying on with Liz to help look after Mum but my sister had hardly slept for a month and our reinforcements were too far away. Day in, day out, with no end in sight, it just felt too hard.

The Wellington sisters persuaded the retirement village to admit Mum to its hospital wing until she could be formally assessed. On our final night in Hastings, I lay in bed and prayed she'd die in her sleep before she knew what we were going to do to her. The following morning Pat and I put her in our car to take her away from Liz's outstanding care and deliver her into the hands of strangers. Sitting in the front seat, Mum sagged over the seatbelt and couldn't — or wouldn't — lift her head to say goodbye. It was 19 January 2009, her fifty-seventh wedding anniversary.

CHAPTER TWENTY-SIX

FORTISIP

ON THE WAY back to Wellington, we stopped to pick up Rose, who was holidaying at Waikanae; she'd offered to help me settle Mum into hospital: TGFS. It took two of us to get Mum into Rose and Mike's beach house where she ate nothing and said little. I registered their shock; I'd forgotten how much she'd deteriorated since her fall.

It was early evening when we arrived at the village. At reception, Rose and I asked for a wheelchair for Mum who was struggling to stand. Instead of heading towards the upmarket studios, we got in the lift and pressed the button to the hospital on the first floor: there was no star beside it.

Silently we pushed Mum's wheelchair down a long corridor obstructed by trolleys spilling over with linen and cleaning products. Her room, one of 60, was tiny compared with her studio, with a view of the carpark instead of the harbour. We put her few clothes in the wardrobe, spread her mohair rug over the single bed and plumped up her special pillow. There was no chair for her to sit in. When we asked for one, staff wheeled in an ugly brown corduroy La-Z-Boy that was too high and missing its footrest.

Mum refused food and drink and our forlorn fussing. We got her into her pyjamas, dispensed her night-time pills, kissed her goodbye, told the staff we were available 24/7 and hoped someone would comfort her when we'd gone. Not ready to leave each other — or Mum — we found ourselves outside her studio. In spite of her month's absence, the door was unlocked. Inside seemed like an oasis of sweet memories, already part of the good old days.

Feeling like gatecrashers, we pulled the last bottle of wine from the fridge and set a half-eaten box of Griffins sampler biscuits on the coffee table between us. As the orange sky faded to black, we curled up in armchairs that smelled of Mum and got loud and emotional at an impromptu farewell party while the guest of honour lay alone on another floor. We were Pip'n'Rose again. Two little girls. Unable to be with our mother, unable to be without her.

WHEN I RETURNED the next day for Mum's health assessment, her pallor was ghostly and she could barely raise her head off her chest. Without a footrest, her feet dangled from the La-Z-Boy in a way I knew would be playing havoc with her back. Even when the care coordinator arrived — usually Mum's cue to buck up — she murmured that she needed help with everything and drifted off to sleep. The coordinator watched her for a few minutes, then beckoned me into a side room.

'Can you come back when she's feeling better?' I asked.

She patted my shoulder. 'I don't need to come back.'

At that moment, I understood that Mum was dying, although the coordinator's report is more upbeat. It notes a gradual decline in her condition but says her need for hospital rather than rest home care is associated with her fractured humerus, and that she 'has the potential to improve as her arm heals'.

We brought paintings over from Mum's studio. In my mind's eye, they remained stacked behind her door, adding to the clutter but comforting us that she wasn't there to stay. Except that may not have been the case. 'Rose has done a great job setting up Mum's room with some of her knick-knacks, and getting the maintenance man to put up pictures on the walls,' I emailed three days after she moved in. Reader, beware.

In the same email, I said Mum had been found lying on her side on the floor of the bathroom attached to the empty room opposite, her second fall since she'd arrived. She seemed unhurt but no one could tell us how long she lay there. After that, staff put a sensor mat by her bed but it was easily tripped by others in the cramped room and was mostly turned off.

I also noted that 'the hospital manager still hasn't come near us or phoned us. It means we haven't had a proper introduction to the hospital or any idea of the care we can expect for Mum. All pretty hopeless, and we will insist on a meeting if she doesn't front up tomorrow.'

When Mum began to get cranky again, demanding to know why she was in hospital and when she could leave, we knew she was rallying. You never knew how you'd find her: dressed or in her pyjamas, bright or agitated, sitting in her oversized chair or curled up on the bed stricken with pain and nausea. Taking her out became almost impossible. She was terrified of falling, reluctant to use the walker with her bad shoulder and uncomfortable in the wheelchair.

Her studio friends came to visit. I wheeled her into a public space where there was room for them to gather round. But Mum soon tired of their gossip, as if their vigour and freedom were an affront to her frailty. It was hard to believe a month earlier she'd been among them.

Mum still couldn't swallow anything more textured than a

smoothie, and even thin fluids made her cough. The cocktail of drugs, to which the GP had added codeine, aggravated her empty stomach. A speech therapist examined her and said there was nothing wrong with her swallowing reflex and her slurred speech was probably a dry mouth from dehydration. I don't remember her linking Mum's difficulties to advancing dementia but there's a query in her notes. This too has a name: dysphagia.

The hospital's answer to Mum's eating woes was Fortisip, a milk-based protein supplement that she detested. To me, the small foil-lined boxes represented everything that was wrong with the place. Whenever I visited, there'd be two or three in various stages of deterioration, oozing warm, sweet liquid through a hole in the top, out of which poked a sticky straw. The boxes, which seemed to me to be a breeding ground for bugs, were never refrigerated. They were meant to be thrown out after 24 hours of being opened but no one ever recorded the date on them. 'Old people can live on a box of Fortisip a day,' the GP said ominously. I weighed one in my hand and tried to work out how many sips Mum had taken out of it.

One lunchtime, I overrode her protests and wheeled her to the dining room. We both needed a change of scene. She might meet someone she liked, I said. As soon as we walked in, I regretted making her come. Some people are able to bring warmth and ease to these situations. I'm not one of them; I had no more idea how to relate to Mum's doddery tablemates than she did.

The only people talking were the staff, some with just the right tone and manner, others loud and patronising. One of them put a plate of grey purée in front of Mum, who met the 'Come on, Rosaleen, eat up,' with narrowed eyes and pursed lips. I wheeled her out before her silent protest turned to downright rudeness.

'Let's share an Eskimo Pie,' I said when we got back to her room. I'd left some in the communal freezer.

'Shall we?' She leaned in as if I'd suggested we play hooky, which in a way I had.

I returned with the ice cream and two spoons, and she made a show of eating a couple of mouthfuls.

'One more?' I said, attacking my end in solidarity.

She waved her hand in front of her face like a papal blessing. '*Uh-uh*. Big lunch.'

IT BECAME CLEAR that Mum was never going back to her studio even if her shoulder did heal. The pressure went on us to sell it. As long as it remained vacant, she'd be charged nearly $300 a week, the base rate for studio care she was no longer receiving, on top of $842 a week for hospital care of arguably dubious quality. The hospital notes I requested later are more detailed and personal than Mum's studio notes, a sad litany of her anxiety and confusion, dominated by the word 'refused': to shower, to get up and dressed, to take her medication — above all, to eat.

The notes don't mention the day Rose found Mum sitting soiled in her chair. 'It took 15 minutes to get any assistance by which time I had done my best for her in a bathroom minus any cleaning items (1 small, yellow hand towel) and no means to fill the small basin,' she emailed. 'There was tension among the staff, particularly at hand-over time — i.e. whose responsibility exactly was it? It raised for me again very starkly — is this the place I want Mum to be?'

Nor do they mention the failure to maintain a food and fluid chart, although the need for one is recorded twice. 'If the hospital's concern is primarily about Mum's eating, it's not clear what they are really doing about it,' Rose emailed. 'The top page on the chart today was dated 2/02/09 and had one entry — *few sips of juice at lunchtime.* The rest of the page was entirely bare — and that was 2 days ago. Mum was mellow and sadly aware. I read to her for ages and brushed her hair. I agree she is very frail though she has surprising use of her left arm and shoulder.'

We'd had doubts about Mum's care in her studio. Now she couldn't walk, toilet or feed herself without help. Most staff did their best but they seemed bemused by her obstruction, too stretched to provide more than basic care and react to crises. Management seemed invisible. Real estate not health care.

Spurred on by Rose's email, I rang another retirement village. The hospital manager told me they had an unexpected vacancy. I raced around before she changed her mind. Walking in the front door, I felt myself breathe again. It was quiet, orderly, a world away from where Mum was stranded. The room the manager showed me was big and airy, marred only by a lingering smell in the bathroom.

I don't know why she let us jump the queue but it was no time for manners and I accepted on the spot, knowing my sisters felt as desperate as I did. Three weeks after Mum left Hastings, Ginny and Kate packed her things again and said goodbye to a few special staff and her studio buddies at the old village. On the way out, they picked up a complaint form. Consumed in our own life-and-death drama, we never filled it in. We just took Mum away and put that place behind us.

In retrospect, I might have thought that our low opinion of the care Mum received there was skewed by our personal grief about her illness, that our standards were simply too high. But in 2013 the brave daughter of a rest home resident in the same village did make an official complaint after she found her mother, who'd had a stroke and suffered from Alzheimer's disease, covered in her own faeces three times.

A Ministry of Health spot audit upheld the daughter's concerns and criticised the care given to all hospital and rest home residents there. It echoed our own misgivings about the studios as well: that complaints weren't always registered, care plans were inadequate, communication between staff broke down between shifts, and clinical leadership was not evident. The audit also noted the absence of an infection control team in the rest home, reminding me of the two norovirus outbreaks during Mum's studio stay. The village manager resigned.

Reading this sorry account, I felt vindicated — and regretful. If we'd filled in our complaint form at the time, other residents might have been spared years of suffering. Other families, too.

CHAPTER TWENTY-SEVEN

GOING
HOME

AT NINE IN the morning, I arrived at the new hospital to find Mum dressed and sitting in a chair with a footrest, her hair brushed, looking through her photo albums. Her *Il Divo* CD played softly on the stereo. Beside her was a chilled box of Fortisip. Her voice was croaky but she was calm.

A nurse came to tell me she'd slept well. The manager hovered. The activities officer put her head around the door to say she'd take Mum to meet the other residents that afternoon for 'reminiscing'. The plump cook in the kitchen said, 'Don't worry, we'll fatten your Mum up,' and I almost believed her.

Mum's GP called in. When he asked her to walk, she got up out of her chair by herself — something her left shoulder usually stopped her from doing — and shuffled once around the bed with the walker before refusing to go any further. The GP removed her anti-nausea medication and codeine, and said he'd like to see her off all her drugs. I told him we had to make a family decision about Aricept. On the internet, I'd found stories of some people's parents who were calmer — perhaps less aware — after stopping it, others who'd deteriorated. Whatever we did was going to be a lottery.

The lull was short-lived. For us, the new set-up seemed infinitely better, kinder, more tranquil than the old. But for Mum, it was the same prison, only the cell was bigger and the guards less harried. She showed no interest in the world beyond her room. She fell in the bathroom, escaping with a graze. Most of all, she refused to eat.

Matt came home for the first time since Mum had broken her humerus. After taking his son Fin to visit, he sent an email:

From: Matt
To: Rose; Ginny; Pip; Kate; Liz
Sent: Monday, February 17, 2009 08:24 PM
Subject: Mum

We spent most of Sunday afternoon with Mum. She still seems very unsettled and anxious. I guess I would be too.

I think the lack of mobility (waiting for someone to move her) is biting hard. She was uninterested in working out how to propel herself in the wheelchair. I think it would be life-changing if she could see her way clear to start wheeling herself. Methinks the self-image of not being seen to struggle (with something so 'basic') is getting in the way. The night-time walkabouts might be a part of this.

The other big challenge is probably the paucity of potential buddies. She appeared to be denying she has anything in common with the other residents. But that may be a mood thing I hope.

I suspect her days are very long. If her TV is still around, it may not be a bad idea. I tried to get her to put the loose photos in an album — but she wasn't very interested. I will ring the presbytery and see if they have a regular visiting schedule.

We tried to take her out for a walk/wheel. She was very keen until we got outside, then complained bitterly about the 'wind' — all 0.5 knots of it.

She seemed most at ease when we simply sat. I will start taking my computer up to her room, and just be around. Maybe we could all take things we need to do.

All rather sad really. Mum has moved into the next phase physically, but her mind and will are still 3 chapters back. Will be back there today.

Matt

This is the final email in the trail of thousands that recorded our five-year saga of looking after Mum. There were no words for what came next: there was just the being there. Ginny, in bed with a sore throat, pined that she couldn't be. I too bowed out for the weekend to bring the gang women together for one last time before my book was published. This gathering, at our house, was even more fractious than the one where they'd agreed to go ahead.

The time for consultation was coming to an end. Quick decisions had to be made about everything from the title and cover photo to the book launch and division of royalties. Everyone was edgy. No one appreciated my mother was dying. As the women left, my son Liam's girlfriend Aurora arrived from California to meet our family for the first time and found herself pressing noses in a hongi in the kitchen.

Mum's brother Des flew in from Adelaide and came to stay as well. I hoped his company might soothe Mum but after going to see her alone, he came back shaken, less seasoned than the rest of us. After that we went together in short bursts; it was too hard to stay long.

Each day Mum's rage burned brighter as her body dimmed. A passionate, feral rejection of any kind of nourishment took hold. 'Yuk,' she'd screech, spitting ice cream over the luckless person who tried to spoon it into her mouth. She spat out Fortisip. Spat out her pills. Spat out the toothpaste when staff tried to clean her teeth. Some deeper knowing seemed to fuel the resistance that burned her up like a fire, leaving her with hardly the strength to draw a sip of water up a straw.

You might get a sweet smile when you arrived or sometimes a wry one as if to say, *Ah, so you've finally come to see me.* But almost at once her face would darken and her voice become shrill: 'Get me out of here. How long do I have to stay? I want to go home.'

'Do you think she means Wadestown Road?' asked a rare visitor from the outside world.

'No,' Mum wailed through colourless, cracked lips that revealed her toothless gap.

'I think she's talking about Roxburgh,' said Liz. Mum's old photos were the only thing that calmed her, though she could no longer recite the names of her 29 classmates.

Desperate to distract her one afternoon, Des and I wheeled her to the day room where a young woman played golden oldies on a guitar. Mum had sung along the week before, Rose said. But while the other residents smiled and swayed, Mum rolled her eyes and hissed 'Boring' until we were forced to take her out. Anything that smacked of fake cheer infuriated her. 'Pssshhhh!' she'd say — or 'Shut up!' — if she thought we were getting sentimental.

'I want to go home,' she shouted as we put on our jackets.

'Tomorrow, Mum, we'll take you home tomorrow,' I said in a last-ditch attempt at therapeutic fibbing.

'That's another nine hours. I want to go now.'

In the carpark, Des and I were both in tears. 'I won't be coming back for the funeral,' he said. 'We don't come back for funerals.'

Mum's grandchildren could still get through her defences. As she shooed Matt away one day, he heard her say, 'I love Fin.'

One evening, 25-year-old Liam offered to visit on his own. I could see he was anxious and suggested he get out her photo albums, although she'd begun accusing us of trying to distract her if we tried that. He came back beaming. Mum had been in bed when he arrived. He knelt beside her and they went through the albums while she told him stories about her family. A carer put her head round the door and asked if they'd like supper. When the carer left, Mum leaned into Liam. 'She'll probably think we're dating,' she said.

The quip went round the family: some light relief.

Liz came down from Hastings. 'I want to go home,' Mum shouted as we kissed her pinched cheeks yet again and went to leave. I gave my sister a helpless look. Our eyes locked. Suddenly we knew what to do.

Liz sat down again and stroked Mum's hand. 'You can go, Mum,' she said. 'It's OK.'

Mum stopped tugging at the mohair rug over her knees. 'When? When can I go?'

I glanced at Liz and she nodded. 'Now, Mum,' I said. 'You can go now.'

'Yes,' Liz said. 'Go to Dad. We'll be all right.'

Mum's shoulders slumped. 'I *miss* him.'

'Yes.' I named her older brother Gerard. Liz added other family and friends who were no longer alive. She could go to them too, we said.

A frown came over Mum's face as she considered the list. 'They're all *dead*,' she said at last.

We took a deep breath. 'Yes.'

Her eyes closed. 'Can I?' An exhalation more than a question.

'Yes, Mum. Just go.' I couldn't believe it had taken us so long to understand. She knew what she needed to do; we were the ones who hadn't been able to bear her message.

STILL MUM DIDN'T GO. Over the weekend she was raw and angry again. On Sunday Des took the early morning flight back to Adelaide. He wouldn't let me drive him to the airport but I got up before dawn to make him a cup of tea and found him reading by torchlight at the kitchen table, as if the electric light could possibly disturb our sleep at the other end of the house. It was such a Mum thing to do — once upon a time — not wanting to be a bother. I snuggled up beside my 73-year-old uncle, the next best thing to her.

'Careful,' he said. 'People will probably think we're dating.'

That afternoon Mum was more agitated than ever. When nothing would calm her, I asked the staff to give her a sedative. The GP would have to prescribe it, they said. In the three years Mum had been his patient, it was the first time we'd needed his help outside normal hours. The message came back that he wasn't available.

On Monday morning, Liz drove home to Hastings. Although I'd agreed to see Mum first thing, I hung out washing, checked emails and put off having to face her alone. When I got there, the manager was sitting with her. Later, I thanked her.

'If I was like that, I wouldn't want to be on my own,' she said.

I bristled at the reproach, real or imagined. *We've been at Mum's side for years,* I wanted to shout. *It's too hard, we can't do it any more.*

After I left, Mum was given an enema, Paracetamol suppositories, and Clonazepam liquid for her agitation, prescribed by the GP without seeing her. A hospice nurse also visited. I know these things because they're recorded in the hospital notes.

After being prescribed more Clonazepam in the late afternoon, still without having seen the GP, Mum sank into semi-consciousness. Around seven, he finally appeared at her door.

From her chair by Mum's side, Rose asked him if he would expect the drug to have that effect. His look of shock was all the answer we needed. He held his briefcase in front of him like a shield and made no attempt to come closer. We were glad; we didn't want him anywhere near our mother.

Liz had just got inside her house when we rang to say Mum was worse. 'I'm on my way,' she said, turning around and driving back to Wellington. Des, who'd touched down in Adelaide 24 hours earlier, caught the next plane back too: our kaumatua needed us as much as we needed him.

With the support of the staff, our extended family took over the visitors' lounge close to Mum's room. All six of her children were present, and most of theirs. We took it in turns to sit with her. When it was my turn, I claimed the blue foot-stool near her face and surveyed its ravaged landscape: the high mound of her forehead, the peaks of her cheekbones, the gullies of her eye sockets, the tight plane of her jaw.

'Are you holding her hand?' Matt said.

'Yes.'

'Don't let go.'

As if.

From time to time, two Filipina nurses came in and swabbed Mum's mouth and checked her pulse with exquisite tenderness, then left us to our farewells. Mum's breathing became shallower. I asked if we should get the others.

Kate, our own nurse, explained the stages of breathing before death. For a few minutes more, we watched Mum's chest rise and fall, the gap lengthen between each rattly intake of air. 'Maybe I will,' she said.

People filed into the dimly lit room and spilled out into the corridor. I'd felt cheated when, after weeks of sitting by his bed, Dad died alone, as if he couldn't leave us while we were watching. Not so, Mum. Our life giver and matriarch, our compass and nemesis drew her family around her like a cloak. I knew I should give up my place at her head but I pressed my face into the bedcover and hung on to her hand, still the strongest part of her. Trying to warm it with my own. Waiting for some small pressure in return. As always, needing more from her than she was able to give me.

'We are a tableau,' Rose's husband Mike said, putting the sacred into words.

'She can't go, she hasn't appointed a successor,' Kate said. Laughter filled the room then died away as she added, 'Who will hold us together now?'

In the silence, broken only by Ginny's quiet sobs, we contemplated the awe and mystery of our mother's passing. And yet, when the final moment came, it was so ordinary. Just Mum lying there. Just her breath, fainter and fainter. Nothing to distinguish life from death except endless space where the next breath should have been.

At 10.50 p.m. on Monday, 23 February 2009, Rosaleen Mary Desmond née Waigth, aged 79, went home.

EPILOGUE

AFTER MUM DIED, I did what I couldn't do while she was alive: I took her in. As her casket edged through our kitchen door, the startled repairman with his head in the dishwasher turned the colour of his whiteware. We laid Mum out in the small room in the centre of our house, as hallowed as a chapel with its pink-tiled fireplace, leadlight windows and oregon wood panelling. Photos of Dad and Pat's parents, also dead, looked down from the mantelpiece.

Liz, who'd kept a vigil all night at the hospital, had dressed Mum in a buttoned taupe cardigan and high-necked top that hid the wrinkles she hated, applied a bright red lipstick and tucked a flower between her hands. The casket's white satin lining brought colour to Mum's cheeks. She looked better than I expected. Most of all, she was peaceful.

Each night Liz reapplied the lipstick and covered Mum's face with a muslin cloth so her skin wouldn't dry out. Before I went to bed, I'd fold the cloth down: a body could suffocate under there. Each morning Mum looked softer somehow, as if the strain of her ordeal was departing with her spirit. I was so grateful it was over. But there was a numb, tearless place in my heart where my love should have been. People said my mother had been gone a long time, that I'd already done my grieving. I feared I hadn't even begun.

Of those four days with Mum under our roof, I only recall fragments: casseroles appearing as if by magic to feed the swag of family drawn to the Irish-style wake; Mum's teenage grandkids swapping beers and yarns around our brick barbecue late into the night; Eva Cassidy's soulful lament about lost love playing on the stereo just as the funeral director arrived to take Mum away for the last time; my cousin and his wife returning with water from their stream to bless the house afterwards.

On the last night, we held a vigil at St Anne's in Newtown where for years Mum had done the cleaning, arranged the flowers and gone to Mass. We took her with us, of course — the younger grandchildren perched around her in the hearse — and placed her casket in front of the altar, though she'd have been happier down the back. She'd have shied away from the attention too: the stories and songs and memories in her honour.

Liz acknowledged the last hard years in a poem she'd written, a lovely thing that ended with the lines, 'There in the glass, I see your look / Your gentle, empty stare. / You close your eyes. I close your book / And stand and brush your hair.'

Mostly, though, we remembered Mum the way she used to be. One of Dad's brothers said the first time Dad took his young love home, she was like sunshine coming into their house. Liam said she had a way of making each grandchild feel like the only person in a crowded room. Our friends praised her cooking and her listening ear. A neighbour from Wadestown said she'd never forget the compassionate, loyal friend she called Florence Nightingale.

I had no words to express my own feelings but Matt persuaded me to read from my book that Mum would never see in print. I chose a passage about borrowing her vacuum cleaner to try and bring order to our women's house, and my efforts to retrieve the metal pipe after one of the Black Power boys commandeered it. The moral of the story: I'd rather offend any number of gang members than upset my mother.

At the requiem Mass the next morning, Rose's husband Mike reminded the full church of 'the Roxburgh girl, the doctor's wife, the mother of six, the elegant woman of extraordinary grace and kindness, the dream grandmother and great-grandmother. The homemaker. The mother to so many. The lover of people and fun. The private sufferer. The woman of constancy and compassion.'

Afterwards, Mum's children linked hands around her closed casket in a private farewell. Then Matt took over. 'I've had a chat with Mum,' he told us. 'She says it is enough now. She says it has been a little too much fuss. She'd like us to start paying more attention to each other.' He suggested we take a rose from the wreath on Mum's casket to remember her by, then find the door and walk out into the sunshine.

TEN MONTHS LATER, I was still looking for the door. Matt, back for Christmas, had persuaded us to bury Mum's ashes while he was home. I wasn't ready for this final goodbye. Everything felt jangly and disorganised. No one had taken charge. He had to lead the graveside ceremony, I told him; I wouldn't be able to say anything.

That morning I woke from a dream that I'd followed a group of people into a thick forest and had no idea how to get back. Then it was my birthday. I began eating a huge pavlova like the ones Mum used to whip up. I stopped scoffing it long enough to ask a woman if she wanted some. 'No,' she said. 'You eat a whole lot but you're still not satisfied.'

I could hear Pat whistling in the kitchen. Outside, the northerly banged against the house. It hadn't let up all night; I knew because I'd been awake for most of it. I got out of bed to make Coronation Chicken, Mum's signature party dish. As I chopped and fried and stirred, I kept thinking of a fable I'd read in Clarissa Pinkola Estés's *Women Who Run With the Wolves*.

'Vasalisa the Wise' is the tale of a young woman whose 'too-good' mother dies, leaving her a tiny doll. When Vasalisa's father remarries, her stepmother and stepsisters banish her into the forest to find fire. The doll guides her to the hovel of the old hag, Baba Yaga, who sets her impossible household tasks such as separating poppy seeds from dirt (that the doll helps her complete), then sends her off with a fiery skull on a stick to light her way. It is the skull of intuition, the wild woman 'blaze of knowing' that, on Vasalisa's return home, burns her tormentors to cinders.

All morning the story nagged at me in ways I didn't understand. By the time we got to the Karori Cemetery, the wind had brought misty rain in its wake. We parked our cars and filed through the damp grass, as bedraggled as any band of orphans. At the end of a row of graves, we gathered around a concrete slab edged by trees that bowed and sighed as if they, too, were in mourning. When Dad was dying, Mum had discovered his mother was buried there in an unmarked grave and had erected a black marble tombstone to them both. Now her name appeared below theirs.

Matt welcomed the family members who'd braved the gale. Liz read her poem again. Rose dug two holes with her trowel: one to plant a cyclamen, as Mum would have done, and one for her ashes. Kate linked arms with Ginny as they mopped their eyes. I stood mute and miserable, my mind filled with the image of Mum's skeletal face in death. Reluctantly I joined the line to dip her long-handled silver spoons into her engraved silver urn and watch the crumbly dust — all that remained of her — drizzle into the earth and scatter on the wind.

Just as people began to move away, leaving me marooned in silence, my heart cracked open. Out poured my garbled thoughts on a flood of pent-up tears. Something about dementia having unleashed the wild woman in Mum. Confronted by her illness, her spirit rebelled and became fierce, as it had to. This fierceness was her essence, not an aberration. Mum wasn't two people, one before and another after she got dementia. The disease robbed her of almost everything but it freed her intuition.

After a lifetime of being good and quiet, Mum demanded to be seen and heard. Imprisoned in the unbearable isolation of forgetting, she shed her restraint and clamoured for connection. When all else failed, she had to choose between staying with us and going home. To end her suffering — and ours — she walked the path of starvation alone, an act of great courage and love. Mum had picked up her wild woman torch and passed it on, I said. It was up to us to keep it alight. Men, too, since every wild woman needs a wild man.

My family let me finish. There were tears. Hugs. More wild woman stories. Liz's husband, Dave, an inveterate speedster, said Mum had urged him to put his foot down in his red Daimler Dart when he took her for a spin during the dementia years. I pictured her wearing sunglasses and a scarf like Grace Kelly, her eyes shining, her face flushed in the wind.

It struck me that my dream and the story of Vasalisa were telling me the same thing. Dementia had led me deep into unknown territory. I, too, had to find the mother beneath the too-good one whose sweet pavlova was never going to be enough to sustain me. This new mother was a fearsome teacher who tried me sorely before handing over the glowing torch of intuition. Armed with her gift, there was nothing else to do but descend into my soul and sing over her ashes. To honour her life. To understand her suffering. To begin making my own way home.

This is my song for her.

BIBLIOGRAPHY

Bryden, Christine. (2015). *Before I Forget: How I Survived a Diagnosis of Younger-Onset Dementia.* Sydney: Penguin Books Australia.

Carroll, Lewis. (1865, 2015). *Alice's Adventures in Wonderland.* London: Pan MacMillan.

Estés, Clarissa Pinkola. (1992). *Women Who Run With the Wolves: Contacting the Power of the Wild Woman.* London: Rider, Random House.

Fadiman, Anne. (1997). *The Spirit Catches You and You Fall Down: A Hmong Child, Her American Doctors, and the Collision of Two Cultures.* New York: Farrar, Straus and Giroux.

Gawande, Atul. (2014). *Being Mortal: Illness, Medicine, and What Matters in the End.* London: Profile Books Ltd.

Gellhorn, Martha. (1979, 2001). *Travels with Myself and Another.* London: Penguin.

Gornick, Vivian. (2001). *The Situation and the Story: The Art of Personal Narrative.* New York: Farrar, Straus and Giroux.

Grant, Susannah. (2017). *Windows on a Women's World: The Dominican Sisters of Aotearoa New Zealand.* Dunedin: Otago University Press.

Magnusson, Sally. (2014). *Where Memories Go: Why Dementia Changes Everything.* London: Two Roads, Hodder & Stoughton.

Maté, Gabor. (2003). *When the Body Says No: Understanding the Stress-Disease Connection.* New York: John Wiley & Sons.

ACKNOWLEDGEMENTS

WRITING ABOUT MUM would not have been possible without the support of my sisters Liz, Rose, Ginny and Kate, and our brother Matt. I am indebted to them (and their families) for the joint care of Mum after she got dementia; for sharing their emails, memories and feedback on drafts of this book; and for trusting me to honour Mum's life despite feeling conflicted about her privacy and the privacy of our family. I am forever grateful for their love and understanding as I strove to tell my version of events that affected us all.

The support of Mum's brother Des means more than he can know. Much of the material about Mum's Roxburgh childhood and her ancestors comes from a conversation I recorded with him and Mum on the cusp of her illness, and subsequent discussions. I've also drawn on my brother-in-law Mike Fitzsimon's eulogy at Mum's funeral, Eileen Binns' meticulous research of Waigth family history, and historical Roxburgh resources. The Hocken Library solved the mystery of 'maori heads' (snow tussock) mentioned in my great-grandmother's obituary.

My deepest appreciation goes to Garry Cockburn, who helped me find Mum as I was losing her to dementia. Fiona Kidman's memoir-writing course got me started putting words on the page. Rebecca Lancashire gave me the idea for a new first chapter. Mandy Hager and Alison Parr read drafts and provided vital encouragement.

Dementia advocates Mary Slater, Frances Blyth, Anne Schumacher and particularly educator Emma Fromings enhanced my knowledge of the disease and its effect on families. Alzheimers Wellington, led by Carol Day, was a rare beacon when we were caring for Mum, as was the Chelsea Club, whose then manager Barbara Reddish and staff deserve our deepest gratitude.

The responsibility of writing about real people weighs heavily on me. I have named Mum's family and some of her special friends, including Lorna, Rosemary, Jeanette, Margaret, Lesla, Marie, Mark and David. However, the names of carers and health professionals have been changed or omitted to protect their identity.

I've drawn on the wisdom of a number of other writers who are acknowledged in the bibliography. They, and many other people, have contributed to my insights about dementia, ageing and life. I am grateful to you all.

A big thank you to my publisher Nicola Legat for backing me again, along with her dedicated team at Massey University Press: Anna Bowbyes, Sarah Thornton, Emma Neale and Kate Barraclough. It takes a village to raise a book.

My husband Pat steadied me with his unwavering belief in me and this story. He is my first and most constant reader, and my lifelong companion. My children and grandchildren lit up Mum's life as they light up ours. Special thanks to my daughter Megan for her careful reading of the final draft.

Dad, a background figure in this book, was pivotal in my life and in Mum's. Together they raised our family with love and care, and made me who I am.

My final thanks go to Rosaleen Desmond née Waigth. I hope you can forgive me for putting you centre stage, Mum. All I can say is that you deserve to be there.

ABOUT THE AUTHOR

PIP DESMOND is a Wellington writer, editor and oral historian. She is the author of the award-winning *Trust: A True Story of Women and Gangs* and *The War That Never Ended: New Zealand Veterans Remember Korea*. Pip has an MA in creative writing and runs communications company 2Write with her husband Pat. They have three children and four beautiful grandchildren.

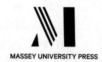

MASSEY UNIVERSITY PRESS

For more information about our books please visit
www.masseypress.ac.nz